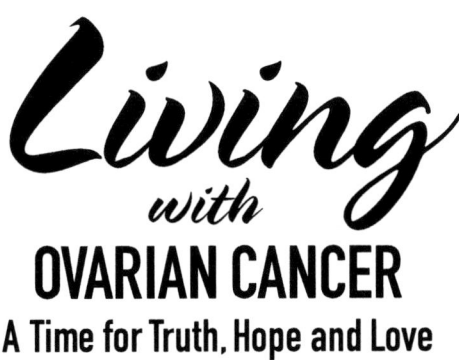

Living
with
OVARIAN CANCER
A Time for Truth, Hope and Love

Nina Davidson Arnold

Living with Ovarian Cancer
A Time for Truth, Hope and Love

by Nina Davidson Arnold

Library of Congress Control Number: 2003096555
ISBN 0-9745355-0-8

First Printing – October 2003

Additional copies of this book are available by mail:
Send $12.00 for each copy (includes tax and postage) to:
Nina Davidson Arnold
Living with Ovarian Cancer
P.O. Box 51
Johnston City, IL 62951-0051

Wholesale inquiries welcome.

Printed in the USA by:

Morris Publishing
3212 East Highway 30
Kearney, NE 68847
1-800-650-7888

Dedication

This book is lovingly dedicated to my husband, Dennis; my son, Anthony; and my daughter-in-law, Aimee. Without their continuous love, encouragement and assistance, I would not have had the strength or perseverance to live through these five-and-a-half years or to finish this manuscript. My family is indeed the most precious gift of life.

Acknowledgements

There are numerous individuals whom I would like to acknowledge and thank for their part in supporting me as I worked on this book and are as follows:

My husband, Dennis, who suggested that I summarize my journals and continuously encouraged me to finish the work to share with other cancer patients.

My son, Anthony, and daughter-in-law, Aimee, who were helpful with suggestions and were responsible for publishing the manuscript.

My sisters, Lola Riley and Kasey Rueffer, who were consistent in their loving concerns for my well-being when I needed it most.

My lifetime friend, Beverly Faaborg, who encouraged me with technical assistance, tireless efforts, perseverance and insistence that this journal be published.

Joe and Stephanie Sacco, who offered additional assistance with the final review of the manuscript, and design and printing of this book.

My two oncologists, all my doctors, and many nurses, who gave me expert care and support during the various stages of my illness.

My special friends, who offered their gifts of love, prayers, encouragement and support, which inspired me to prevail.

And finally a special thanks to everyone who dedicated their time and effort to the laborious task of continually reviewing and proofing this book. Your help was greatly appreciated.

Foreword

A Time for Truth, Hope and Love – A Son's Reflections

I think it has been said that the truly unexpected things in life happen on a Tuesday afternoon, and so it was when we found out that my mother was diagnosed with ovarian cancer in 1997.

Like the thousands of others diagnosed with cancer, my mother had become a statistic. Almost everyone has at least one relative or close friend that is living with cancer. Over the last five years several of my friends and peers have had loved ones with various forms of cancer, many are survivors in spite of their cancer, still willing and able to fight. From the perspective of a family member, the phases of shock, realization, coping, and acceptance of the disease along with the confusion of drug names and treatments, and a feeling of hopelessness, only increased the stress of the situation for everyone involved. My mother was willing to fight and our family was willing to do anything possible to help her...and the fight against cancer consumed all of us.

I was blessed with loving, supportive parents who have always been there, through successes and failures, to help me back up and challenge me to continue on, conquering my fears and obstacles. More than anything, I wanted to return this love and support, especially during my mother's fight with cancer. It crushed me emotionally, spiritually, and physically to see my mother's health deteriorate just a little more each time I saw her. There was no bridge I could build, no treatment I could recommend, and no quantifiable help I could provide. The cancer had tied my frustrated hands to offer my mother only my support, time, and love.

From an emotional vantage point, I wondered how this could happen, why was I not chosen instead of my fragile mother to be inflicted with this disease that requires strength and determination to survive? After all, if my God was also just, loving, and looked after his true angels of the earth, how could he inflict such pain on such a loving innocent person of devout faith? In truth, my mother has exhibited a Herculean strength and will-to-live through it all, which would surpass anything I would possibly be able to endure. My father has been a never-resting fortress and foundation to my mother, surrounding, supporting, and protecting her with love and companionship.

After almost six years, I now look at my mother as an amazing person beating the odds with each passing minute, a person who inspires others with hope, and proves the importance of living every moment to its fullest.

When my mother committed herself to writing this book, she did it in hopes that publishing her experiences would not only help those directly dealing with cancer but would also help caregivers, family, and friends understand the emotional impact and trauma caused by cancer and its treatments.

Anthony Arnold
Summer 2003

Introduction

At my husband's coaxing, I was motivated to publish my memoirs of the five-and-a-half years I have lived with ovarian cancer, stage IV as diagnosed in May of 1997. Ovarian cancer is a chronic disease that can, in many cases, be treated for a long period of time. Stage IV means the cancer has metastasized to other parts of the body. Survival rates vary with different stages of the disease, but may be as much as seven years or more with proper treatment. I would never have visualized the words I am writing or the experiences I have encountered during this time. Over these life-changing years, I retired from my professional life as an artist, prioritized my objectives, learned to live one day at a time, and endeavored to cope with each new experience as a way of life. During this time, I kept detailed journals that recorded medical data, explanations of procedures, side effects from chemotherapy drugs, and problems that occurred following treatments. Notations from these journals reflect the various emotions I felt as I responded to the disease, the impact of chemotherapy, the chronic fatigue, and the need for spiritual consolation. Methods of coping were varied and sporadic. A healthy positive attitude toward coping was always more comforting than the occasional mood of despair.

It is my intention that this chronological account of experiences encountered, and methods by which I coped, be helpful to other women with a similar diagnosis who also face the many challenges of this disease. It is not written to frighten or alarm the cancer patient, but to record honest evaluation of real emotional responses in dealing with the daily problems of the disease. I hope to emphasize that feelings of despair, of hopelessness, and of fright, are normal. I am embarrassed, somewhat, by my own thoughts and some of the emotional outbursts I have made in my journal. Such a wimp, I am! This account bares my soul with many outcries that might best be left unwritten. However, this is an honest account of how I actually felt at various moments during my endeavor to survive. I am grateful that I could still see beauty about me and that I recorded my thoughts in that direction also. It is hoped that only the beautiful thoughts I have had may be most memorable and not my weakness of spirit. The power to experience beauty along the way makes the journey more tolerable. Each step today and into tomorrow can be one of faith and hope. Coping with cancer can mean attempting to live life in spite of an incurable disease – grasping each moment as a gift of time and enjoying every simple pleasure that comes one's way.

Writing has given me the opportunity to look into myself. I found that I could more easily cope with my fears and anxieties by writing about them. Daily writing gave me not only a chronological account of my emotions in progression, but also a record of medical data and procedures that were related to my feelings on a particular day. Following each chemotherapy treatment, an account of side effects, bodily functions, dietary problems, fatigue, and general well being was recorded. From these inclusions, I could predict, to some degree, what might be expected from treatments that followed. Many days I wrote not about my problems, but about simple pleasures of life, beautiful aspects of nature, or things for which I was most thankful. Other days, I recorded notes of fear and desperation. Many notes were taken regarding contacts with health insurance personnel and pre-certification numbers needed for medical procedures. These were helpful for future reference if problems occurred with health insurance claims. For a cancer patient, the importance of keeping a daily journal cannot be overemphasized.

From the beginning of diagnosis, I attempted to become knowledgeable concerning ovarian cancer, the chemicals used to treat it, and the side effects of the treatments. The patient's oncologist and the American Cancer Society can offer pamphlets that explain terminology for drugs and treatment. I highly recommend these valuable resources of information. Knowledge helped me feel I had some control of my own well being and allowed me to be able to communicate more meaningfully with my oncologists. By taking charge of myself, I felt it was possible to "have a life" in spite of an illness. Looking at the disease as a way of life made it easier to cope with each new experience. Taking "one day at a time" inspired me to appreciate that day for what it was – another day of life! It was imperative to maintain a healthy attitude during the initial chemotherapy treatment and the nine additional regimens that followed during the course of five-and-a-half years. A positive attitude made it easier to cope with the daily challenges of this disease.

As a way of introducing myself, the following paragraphs, though rather ordinary, explain who I am. I was raised on a farm in Southern Illinois, a happy little girl surrounded by love from my mother, father, two sisters and maternal grandparents. Our life on the farm was one of contentment and security. Weekend pleasures might include a long trip to Cave-in-Rock State Park for fish fries or a simple picnic in the country, sitting on a quilt enjoying the Sunday afternoon with my parents, sisters, and grandparents. These picnics were special with typical picnic fare of fried chicken, sliced tomatoes, good homemade potato salad, corn on the cob, and of course apple pie. Childhood led into teenage years when I was involved in the usual activities of any 14 to 18-year-old youth – church activities, school clubs, band, chorus, friendships and being Homecoming Queen my senior year. I attended college at Southern Illinois University where I found the man of my dreams, Dennis Arnold. We were married while in college and I selected a major compatible with my personality and life expectations. Art was my chosen area of study with an emphasis in textiles and ceramics.

A lifetime career in textiles, mainly weaving, led to a variety of experiences initiated by a two-year assignment with the Peace Corps in Afghanistan. My husband and I returned to the states in the mid-60's ready to start a family and begin our journey through life. We had made our home in the small Northwestern Illinois town of Kewanee, during the years that we raised our one son, Tony, who is now 33. The next three-and-a-half decades were abundant with life's great adventures – raising a son, enjoying family life, experiencing a career as a fiber artist, and traveling throughout the United States to participate in art shows. As a family, we traveled to local and national art shows almost every weekend from April through November. Our itinerary included shows from Michigan to Tennessee, from Pennsylvania to Indiana, and from Colorado to Virginia. A separate art studio at Lake of Egypt served both as a work place and as a pleasant get-away from our active schedule at home in Northwestern Illinois. Life was busy, hectic, happy, challenging, and productive. Family life was centered on a diversified schedule of our son's piano lessons, church activities, travels, and the combination of two careers – my husband's teaching career and mine as an artist. As the years rolled by, our son attended college and married. Our lovely daughter-in-law, Aimee, made our family complete.

Gradually, in the early 90's, my health began to deteriorate. Fatigue and muscle pain prompted me to seek medical attention with the thought that I might be suffering from fibromyalgia. Two years later, my strength decreased to a level in which I could not comfortably continue to weave. I decided to discontinue weaving and switch to a less exertive type of artwork – fiber and paper collage. With this medium, I created smaller artwork not requiring the physical effort of large tapestries, which I had previously designed for office buildings and private homes. For several years I maintained two art studios, my home studio in Kewanee and the lake studio in Southern Illinois. A few years before my medical problems confronted me, Dennis had retired. We returned to Southern Illinois and built the home of our dreams. I wanted to be near my sisters. We had no inclination of what the years ahead entailed or that it would prove such a blessing to "be back home."

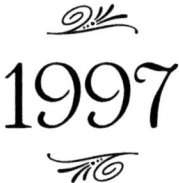

1997

The Year that Changed Our Lives.

The year opened after an enjoyable family Christmas. Tony and Aimee had spent the holidays with us and had returned to their home in Omaha. Dennis and I resumed our normal work schedule at the lake studio. The half-hour drive each morning gave us time to plan the day's schedule. I worked on artwork while Dennis cut mats, framed my artwork and packaged commissioned art pieces for shipment. Each day I found myself groping for strength to design my work and finish it for framing. We worked late and I often fell asleep while Dennis was driving us home.

By May, my appetite had deceased considerably and I could not work in the studio the entire day. On one particular day, I felt a lump in my abdomen. Dennis insisted on immediate medical attention; at which time a CAT scan was given. My doctor disclosed the results of the CAT scan; I had ovarian cancer and surgery was imperative. When my doctor stated those raw and cold words, "you have ovarian cancer – I will arrange for surgery in St. Louis," I reacted with disbelief, despair, and a piercing agony I had never felt before. Our world began to fall apart. We were in anguish – the beautiful love story of our life together, our plans to enjoy my husband's retirement, and our travels were suddenly all at bay. What could we do? What was the future, what was going to happen next? Was there any way out? Attempting to be pragmatic about our anxieties, we decided together to take one day at a time, do what had to be done, and endure the outcome. That seemed to be a more logical approach than surrendering to tears. Actually, the shock was so paralyzing, I could not cry.

I started a journal recording each important piece of information in regard to my disease. Medical notes, appointments, and test results were noted. Confusion made it difficult to concentrate, so I relied on my notes in my daily journal to help me remember and understand what my doctor had told me. Expressions of fear, anxiety and hopelessness, in addition to notations on happiness, joy, moments of thanksgiving, and feelings of wholeness were recorded;

these notes reflected the emotional responses this life-changing drama had created. These daily accounts did not always reflect a pragmatic, logical approach to the predicament in which I found myself, but the words represented my emotions at that time. Sometimes I was very happy and felt I had control of myself; at other times, I found myself in a state of shock with an inability to cope. During the few days while awaiting my initial surgery for removal of the ovaries and the cancer in my abdomen, I had time to reflect and to center my thoughts. I was confused, afraid and extremely anxious about the surgery. My thoughts ranged from fright to thoughts of thanksgiving for my husband and family. The first entry from my journal is recorded below. This and all other entries are dated and indented.

May 24, 1997

I have never had surgery before and am somewhat frightened. I worry that I may not make it out of the operating room. We haven't told our son and daughter-in-law about the cancer surgery yet. This is their anniversary weekend and I don't want to upset them. I have not shed tears and do not know if I will; I know that I have had a very wonderful, full life and am married to the most wonderful husband in the world. He is my strength, confidant, friend, hero, first and only love, and a dependable partner in everything I do. He encourages me in my artwork, he helps me, he takes care of me and he treats me as his most prized possession. I am truly loved and I love him. No one could take his place in my life. We have been blessed with a dear son, Tony, who is sensitive and thoughtful. He is appreciative of what we have given him and for helping him through his Masters degree. He has developed into a responsible young man who is in the prime of forming his life. My daughter-in-law, Aimee, is a treasure. Tall and graceful, she is independent, intelligent, determined and responsible. She is well-organized and makes efficient use of her time. She is a perfect mate for our son. I am blessed. What more could I ask for than all of this – a wonderful husband, son, and daughter-in-law. My two sisters add an extra special blessing to my life. We are good friends and see each other often. All of these joys of life make my life meaningful. I have so much – so much! How can I be sad? After the shock of the bad news and what may face me in the future, I am desperate and so terrified. I do not want to die – there is so much more life that I would like to experience. I am fearful of being in an incompetent state from chemotherapy, in constant pain, and being a burden on Dennis. Fear forces one to cry out to someone – "Help me! Don't leave me! Comfort me!" Dennis reassured me he would be with me always. It is comforting to pray "God don't leave me, be with me as I go through the surgery, stay with me, I want to know You are there. God's Son on earth suffered too, just like common man. He had pain, and maybe dread for His ending mission, but He prevailed. God gives us faith that man, too, can prevail – can accomplish what must be done. It is through this faith in God that I must have the courage to make it through to recovery."

The surgery was 90% successful. The ovaries, fallopian tubes, and uterus were removed (a total abdominal hysterectomy with bilateral salpingo-oopherectomy). Two small areas of cancer could not be removed – a small spot on my liver and a small portion on my diaphragm. This required postoperative chemotherapy. I had been so frightened about the surgery and now another challenge faced me – chemotherapy. I did not know what to expect other than that I would be sick and would lose my hair. My initial treatments of paclitaxel (Taxol) and cisplatin (Platinol) were every three weeks for a six-month regimen. I became quite ill for several days following treatment and lost my hair within the first two weeks. It was important to drink plenty of liquids, mainly water, to help flush the chemicals out of the system and to prevent liver or kidney damage from the drugs. Water prevents dehydration and also aids in preventing neuropathy (nerve damage). I found it difficult to drink liquids or to eat during the few days following chemotherapy. Everything I would take in, I would throw up. Chemotherapy drained my energy level; I found that rest and sleep were imperative. While the side effects of chemotherapy were distressing, I knew that "good days" would eventually follow. During those days, I could do small tasks such as laundry, cooking special dishes, and shopping. Visiting with family and friends was welcomed on those days. We took mini vacations to see Tony and Aimee or short day trips to help maintain the joy of living. In spite of the unpleasant aspects of treatments, I attempted to deal with the disease by enjoying any pleasurable moment that presented itself; I relaxed on the deck, practiced the piano, visited with friends, and spent time in my studio creating artwork. I became involved with any pleasant project, activity, or social event; this helped to prevent boredom and feelings of inadequacy. A feeling of accomplishment and contentment promoted a positive state of mind, a key factor in fighting cancer.

October 13, 1997
Life is like a treasured art piece – its textures and colors, its lines and details. Its spirit is a reflection of the body in which it dwells. Death is a celebration of life and what has been. Without death, there would be no glorious feast at the abundant table of life! Life would not be experienced, beauty would not be seen and music would not be heard. We have nothing to do with being born or being given the opportunity to experience life, but we have everything to do with how we live the life offered to us. We are free to live and in living, we can love, listen, learn, appreciate, and experience all the best that life has to offer. We are a reflection of God who created us. We have the spirit to exemplify beauty, grace, will, love and reflection of God through our lives.

During an illness, one's perspective on life changes, priorities are altered, and relationships become more meaningful. Being surrounded by supportive family members and friends helped to control my anxieties as I shared my concerns with them. I felt a comforting closeness unfold in my relationship to my sisters, Lola and Kasey; there was additional encouragement from my closest friends.

October 24, 1997
My illness has presented time to reflect, to think about what is important and to treasure the moments in life that are most precious. Quality time with my family is highest on the list of priorities. Other special moments include enjoying the simple pleasures of everyday such as hearing the birds sing, admiring a flower, picking ripe tomatoes, helping Dennis mow the grass, cooking a good meal, listening to beautiful music, or reading a get-well message from a friend. Friends who care about me have touched my life in a special way. They have shown it through their cards, letters, phone calls, books, and flowers. It makes me realize how important people are in one's life. I am blessed to have such wonderful friends with each one touching my life in a special way.

In addition to positive reflections, my thoughts turned to self-examination; I questioned my existence. It was distressing that I had become less productive with my artwork, less enthusiastic about keeping my house in order, and certainly less dependable in maintaining social contacts and commitments. My health dictated what I could or could not do. I was troubled that I could not continue creating my artwork to which I had been dedicated; it bothered me greatly to be incompetent in daily chores. It was aggravating that my health problems dictated my social interaction with family and friends.

October 27, 1997
This challenging time of my life has given me time to question my life and purpose. What am I to do with this gift of time? Strength dictates what I can do. Am I to put everything aside and concentrate on helping myself to recovery? Should I continue designing artwork for shows and galleries or give it as a gift to friends and family? Should I take the attitude "whatever will be will be"? (If I truly believed that, I would not be taking chemotherapy.) I feel I must do whatever I can do to help myself. I can use whatever knowledge I possess to get through the problems at hand. We have free choice to react to an illness in various ways. I must do what I can to help myself and when at my lowest point, I can make a request to my Creator for strength beyond understanding.

I continued to create artwork, developing new ideas and art forms for exhibition, sales, and competition. Studio work helped me to be productive and to be involved in something that offered me a feeling of personal achievement. My state of health made it necessary to decrease the number of art shows in which I exhibited.

As Christmas approached, I was apprehensive in planning many holiday activities, as I had to deal with the effects of chemotherapy on a daily basis. Sometimes I became cynical concerning my treatments and failed to focus on the benefits those treatments produced in controlling my disease. While sitting at the infusion center taking chemotherapy, I wrote the following in my journal.

December 9, 1997
This is such a strange way to spend the pre-holiday season. I am sitting here along with two other patients having toxic chemicals infused into my blood stream to kill the

deadly cancer cells in my body. How do we know this
strange and bizarre process will make us better? Perhaps,
sometime, man in the 21st century may find this process
an extremely barbaric one – that of infusing poison into
the body to kill something that is unwanted. At this point,
however, we must trust medical science, the research
available to us, and the doctors whose expert knowledge
makes our efforts in disease control possible.

Following each chemotherapy treatment, there were several days
of side effects. After each cycle of three weekly treatments, I looked forward to two weeks intermission before resuming chemotherapy again.
The side effects were becoming more severe with several days of vomiting, inability to eat, and more time spent in bed. It was advisable to
stay out of crowds to avoid being exposed to a cold or the flu. I was
truly initiated into the peculiarities of chemotherapy with low blood
counts, anemia, and overall weakness. I frequently reassured myself
that these treatments were keeping me alive, giving me more time to be
with my family, and allowing me to fight this disease.

The Christmas holidays were very special. We were most thankful to have this time together with our family. Tony and Aimee flew
home to be with us. We had our traditional Christmas Eve dinner of
chicken and dumplings, opened gifts, and had a humorous photo ses-
sion – some pictures included me without my wig! Aimee had brought
several pairs of huge red paraffin lips to add to the photo fun. Christmas
morning greeted everyone with a large Christmas stocking filled with
goodies. Later in the morning, we traveled to my sister's house for a
family dinner and gift exchange. The evening was robust with over
twenty additional family members meeting at our house for more food
and fun. It was a special year to remember. It was a year that presented
many drastic changes in our lifestyle, and a year that taught us to appreciate each day as a gift of time.

Looking back, I cannot fathom how we managed to continue life on a somewhat normal basis that first year. I had consistent chemotherapy treatments and a multitude of family and friends who came to visit. I cooked meals and entertained, maintained my art studio at the lake, and continued participating in art shows throughout the Midwest. Some weekends, Dennis would represent my work at the shows when I was too sick from chemotherapy to attend. Orders for artwork kept me extremely busy even on days when I had limited energy. On some occasions, I took orders from my bed and had to smile as I thought of doing a booming business from my bedside! We even managed to process garden produce. Dennis renovated the basement into a studio area so that I could create artwork at home instead of driving 30 miles to the lake studio each day. Fortunately, he had retired from teaching and could give me support and help when I needed it. He had planted three acres of grapes in addition to absorbing much of the business aspects of my art studio. We somehow managed to initiate an entirely new way of looking at life.

1998

Beginning the Battle.

During the first six months of treatment, the chemotherapy drugs of Taxol and Platinol were effective in fighting my cancer. A periodic blood test measured a blood protein to determine how well I was responding to chemotherapy. This test measured a tumor marker or cancer antigen (CA-125) produced in the blood as a result of ovarian cancer. A normal value is below 35 U/ml; anything greater indicates cancer cells are active. My serum level was over 900 when I started chemotherapy but decreased to a low of 27 after six months of chemotherapy. In January, unfortunately, my tumor marker began to increase. This meant that my disease was active again – this time in the lymph nodes of my neck. The chemotherapy drugs were losing effect in fighting the disease. Some of the cancer cells were resistant to the treatment and were growing. I became concerned about my life expectancy and what was in store for me.

January 9, 1998
I became "weepy" last night just thinking about the worst this could mean; I am not ready to die just yet – I don't want to leave Dennis alone. Who will find his keys, his daily planner, or his checkbook? He needs help with his diet – who will help him with that?

January 12, 1998
It is always during these four or five days following chemotherapy that I feel so badly and come face-to-face with my mortality. How much time is remaining and what should I do with this precious gift? No answers! Do I continue working – I do not need financial reward but I do need the challenge of creative endeavor and the feeling of accomplishment that results from work. The desire to read music and to play the piano well has always been something I wanted to accomplish. I want to take this goal seriously and accomplish this in my lifetime. Whatever I do, I want to do it better than I have ever done anything in the past.

January 14, 1998

Tired of having no initiative and energy, I want to be well again! I want to be alive again, vigorous and driven. Yes, this is my time to rest but I also want to have energy to do the things I want to do. With energy evading me, it is difficult to feel any degree of vitality.

It was necessary to hire a housekeeper to help with cleaning. This allowed me to use my energy for things I enjoyed doing. Dennis did the final touches to the studio I had designed on the lower level of our home and I sold some of my looms and textile equipment since a low energy level limited my ability to weave.

February 10, 1998

I am so tired again today. I have to force myself to keep going and sometimes feel I will never get well or feel better than I feel right now. My feet are numb and my fingers are beginning to be numb. It is difficult to play the piano and do artwork. My fingernails are thick and hard – I look at my colorless face and feel that I am dying. But then, everyone is dying from the very process of being born and of life itself. We must be wise enough to make each day count. I am putting together sequential thoughts regarding my fight with this health problem. I want to include these ideas in my artwork.

My cancer antigen continued to increase and chemotherapy was discontinued since neuropathy in my hands and feet was becoming severe. Continued use of Taxol could possibly result in leukemia. While waiting to start a new type of treatment, I felt very good since I was not experiencing the side effects of constant chemotherapy.

February 18, 1998

I feel so good! It is wonderful to have this period of time without the side effects of chemotherapy. I pray that my body can be whole again and well from this cancer. If I can help rebuild my body and my immune system can take over, perhaps my own system can fight this thing. God help me!

February 23, 1998

I am feeling so well! I have two more weeks before a second-line of chemotherapy will be determined for me. I pray that the cancer cells are dying and that I will get well. If the cancer antigen stays in the 60's range, it means the disease is stable, yet the count should be lower, closer to 35. Being between first- and second-line treatment puts me in a state of limbo, an anxious state in which I do not know what to expect.

The events of the previous year and my upcoming second-line treatment were wearing on Dennis. He had been under so much stress worrying about me. He sometimes became irritable and upset due to the many responsibilities he faced. That certainly was understandable. He was particularly edgy a few days before I received each antigen result. As the antigen continued to show growth of my disease, I felt I needed to discontinue my artwork and my shows. It was time to start planning my funeral, prepare Dennis to live alone, get the house in order, sell the lake studio, write favorite recipes for our son, and send a letter to dear friends. At the same time, it was also time to enjoy each precious moment together, whether eating breakfast on the deck or enjoying each other's company in lively conversation. My moods of positive and negative thoughts seem to either compliment or cancel each other!

March 8, 1998
Dennis pulled up several articles on ovarian cancer from the Internet to read about new treatments. After receiving results from the cancer antigen a few days ago, I am somewhat discouraged. It has again risen. Much of my emotional energy is expended on hope – hope, prayer, and wishful thinking! I try what I feel may help me such as limiting my sugar, reducing fat consumption, and eating large amounts of vegetables and fruits. Should I give in and admit that nothing is going to make any difference at this point? I have felt so good, as though repair is taking place. It has been two months since my chemotherapy was discontinued; it is imperative that another treatment is started soon. What does this mean? What is hope? For what should I pray? What is my purpose now? My spirit is broken. Is God's purpose made perfect in my suffering? Will God fulfill His purpose in me?

This idea is in Psalm 138:8 –
> *"The Lord will perfect that which concerneth me: thy mercy, O Lord, endureth for ever: forsake not the works of thine own hands."*
> *KJV*

Must I just trust that He will not forsake the work of His hand?

Some days were almost unbearable. Night and day I was obsessed with anxiety concerning my disease. I was comforted in knowing that the body is a miraculous entity capable of healing itself with the vast reservoir of medications available. I believed that miracles are always possible and was encouraged that new drugs were continually being developed. By the end of March, the cancer antigen had more than doubled. I was again in a state of anxiety as I questioned my doctor for options available to me. Cancer in the lymph nodes of my neck had metastasized from the initial ovarian cancer. The malignant lymph nodes were surgically removed and a second-line chemotherapy treatment was initiated; topotecan (Hycamtin) was used for five-days-a-week with three weeks off between cycles. Side effects were not as drastic as those from Taxol – no nausea or vomiting. Neupogen shots were necessary to stimulate white blood cell growth (neutrophils) that fights infection. Dennis learned to give me the required daily injections. Since Neupogen directs all the growth toward white blood cells, platelets can be affected. If the platelets fell below 30, a platelet transfusion was necessary.

As winter bowed its head to allow for the new season, spring seemed to lift the spirit and offer hope. April presented many pleasant moments as I enjoyed the rebirth of spring and visited with my sisters. Each day, there was something to give life meaning.

April 19, 1998
It is a beautiful spring day as I sit on the deck enjoying
the cool crisp air and listening to the singing of the birds.
The cattle in our uncle's pasture South of the deck rest
peacefully under the trees.

My sisters, Lola and Kasey, continually supported me as I shared my health and emotional concerns with them. We shared the highs and lows of my disease, we laughed and cried together, and we enjoyed shopping and attending events in the local area. On one occasion, we spent a memorable day at the Paducah Quilt Show, in Paducah, Kentucky. The show is a national yearly event and features handmade quilts from all over the United States. We met together frequently to enjoy "three sister dinner parties with spouses" every few months. Sometimes the evenings were dressy occasions and sometimes they were casual affairs.

The vineyard that Dennis had started the previous year needed constant care. There was always something to do. He set posts by hand while waiting for his posthole digger to arrive. I helped do easy chores such as tying up grape vines or spreading fertilizer on the plants, usually for very short periods of time. Dennis enjoyed the vineyard, which gave him a reprieve from stress concerning my health. He took a viticulture class at the local college.

In late April, I prepared forty personal letters to my very best friends. I wanted to tell them about my health problem, but most of all I wanted each one to know I valued their friendship, loved them, and treasured the sharing of our lives over the years. Many sensitive responses were returned, which warmed my heart.

Due to inability to continue with my normal workload of artwork and shows, I applied for Disability from the Social Security Administration. It was a difficult decision to admit that I was disabled, unable to do what I used to do, unable to handle art materials as I once did, unable to lift and do heavy work, and unable to do household chores, which I enjoyed. However, unpleasant situations often turned into enjoyable moments by exposing me to a new concept.

April 19, 1998
Hair loss, (alopecia) is to be expected while taking certain types of chemotherapy. This is the second time I have lost my hair. Wigs and hats can make hair loss more tolerable and even fun as the patient explores different head coverings. The fun of hats led to an interesting art project in which I created tiny two-inch miniature hats. Working on the tiny hats makes me happy.

Occasionally I found humor in being bald! No longer did I have bad hair days – I could just pop on a wig and be ready to go. Adding a hat made it even more fun. I always did love hats!

Neuropathy in my hands and feet had to be dealt with daily. I practiced playing the piano, exercised my fingers, and did floor exercises. These efforts did not seem to help, but gave me assurance that I could still manipulate major appendages.

Blood transfusions were required when the hemoglobin count went below 8. This often meant I would be confined to the hospital for four to five hours depending on whether I needed one or two units of blood. During this time, I did a lot of reading.

Each day there was something for which to be thankful – an e-mail from a friend, a call from a former art student, a get-well card from someone at church, a perfect morning drinking coffee on the deck, a visit from family members, or a relaxing dinner by candlelight. Limited energy forced me to select activities carefully. While it was easier to stay at home where I felt safe, I knew that being active was important for me as a cancer patient. It was a challenge to do something out of the ordinary, but I was happier being involved in life than sitting safely at home. My friend, Bev, and I took a two-day tour to Nashville, saw a show, stayed at Opryland Hotel and cruised the Cumberland River on the General Jackson showboat. It was a pleasant trip and not too taxing on my energy reserves.

On several occasions, my sisters spent a few days with me at the lake studio. The relaxing and peaceful environment was soothing and refreshing as we listened to the ripple of the water, enjoyed the lovely scenery, and fished off the dock. We were rewarded with peace and contentment in being together. Nature always presents the opportunity to enjoy one's perfect environment. Afternoon picnics in the back woods at home were a pleasant way to end an active autumn day of chores and appointments. Daily walks in the vineyard kept me active with regular exercise. The many rows of grapevines provided hours of pleasure as I used the vineyard almost daily for short walks. On some days, I used a cane to keep my balance. Neuropathy in my feet made walking more difficult, I found myself having to adjust to a wider gait to maintain my balance.

Limiting stress was a challenge. A daily problem of health insurance notices, incorrect billing, household problems, financial concerns, my husband's well-being and my own problems often prevented me from resting when rest was so necessary.

Swelling in my neck, where the four lymph nodes had been surgically removed in early April, indicated a need for another biopsy. Other lymph nodes were malignant, which required 20 radiation treatments. It was at this point that my doctor felt we must look into the possibility of a stem call transplant. It was during moments of serious decision making that I again turned to my faith.

July 5, 1998

In church this morning, it occurred to me that when one becomes a spirit, one is free. For a split second, I imagined a state of being out of my body. If truly oblivious to physical, emotional, mental responsibilities and necessities of life such as food, shelter, or support from others, one can escape the body and touch into a spiritual world where one is a spirit, not a bodily form. It is difficult to understand, but I think I am beginning to grasp what it might mean. I attempted to meditate today, to relax my mind, to feel the power of faith, and to put my mind into a spiritual form. Without faith, I can do nothing. Faith is the key. If we are made in God's image, we can achieve! We have power to do if we have faith. If I ask, I can receive; I ask for strength and I receive it. As I walked the vineyard, this prayer came into my mind over and over: "God my Creator, grant me strength; may I be a vessel of thy goodness and grace, thy love and understanding? May I pour out to others generously as Thou hast so abundantly poured out to me?"

Early in the summer, my oncologist began to introduce me to the process of a stem cell transplant, which he felt would be beneficial. Without an outside donor, stem cells are removed from the patient and are frozen. The patient is given high dose chemotherapy over several days to kill any remaining cancer cells in the body. After several more days, the cleansed frozen stem cells are injected back into the patient's blood stream; the stem cells activate bone marrow which produces red and white blood cell growth. The complete stem cell transplant process requires about thirty-three days.

Tony and Aimee came home during the summer. This gave us the opportunity to explain the stem cell transplant I was considering. Since the process was not without risk, I needed some encouragement in facing this challenge. They understood the situation and agreed that I should do what my oncologist felt was necessary. After serious concerns were addressed, we enjoyed the remainder of their visit with Tony at the piano playing songs from his studies of classical music.

In late July, I had disturbing news concerning my younger sister's health. She had diagnostic laparoscopic surgery to remove a growth on her ovary. Malignancies were found on both ovaries; it was necessary to do a complete hysterectomy. The diagnosis was ovarian cancer, Stage 1C (microscopic cancer cells). Since the cancer was found in the early stage, there was a 98% chance that she would be cancer free after chemotherapy. I was shaken by the news that my sister was experiencing this dreadful disease, but was thankful it was found in the early onset.

Radiation treatments for the cancer that had again spread to my neck were increased from twenty to twenty-five. While I dealt with the treatments and the hope that they would give me new life, it was comforting to see the vineyard change and flourish. In June of last year, I was not sure I would be alive to visualize the ripe fruit; I was thrilled to not only see grapes on the vines, but also be able to pick some to eat. Dennis continued work on the vineyard, setting posts for new plant rows as I drove the van to each posthole site.

Before starting preliminaries for the stem cell transplant, we took a trip to see Tony and Aimee in Omaha. We toured the Old

Market, sipped coffee at an outdoor café, and ate sushi at a restaurant. We enjoyed every moment with them and included a short visit with friends in Northern Illinois before returning home. My sisters came to encourage me the day before I went to the hospital. We talked of happy moments of childhood and our beloved parents. Such fond memories during our visit helped me feel ready for the stem cell transplant.

The transplant procedure required two days of preliminary chemotherapy a few weeks ahead of the stem cell harvesting process. The drugs cyclophosphamide and cisplatin were used. This was the third type of chemotherapy I had been given. Following the chemotherapy, a catheter was inserted into my chest to allow access to the blood system for the process, injection of drugs, and blood draws. Phereses involves collection of stem cells; these stem cells were then frozen and stored until they were injected back into my body following three or four days of high dose chemotherapy. This dosage is equal to approximately six months of chemotherapy. There was a rest period of three days before my stem cells were infused into my blood system. As my blood counts dropped, there was a need for blood and platelet transfusions to build up white and red blood cells. This stimulated bone marrow production. My sister-in-law coordinated a blood donor program for me. Members of her church and our family were blood donors. Without the support of family and friends, the process I faced would have been much more difficult.

The long duration of hospitalization was not without problems. Low results on a creatinine test required that one of the chemicals, carboplatin, be reduced by 33% to protect my kidneys from damage. The catheter inserted into my chest caused excessive bleeding. Another chemical used, ifosfamide, had to be discontinued one day early because my kidneys could not eliminate the drug quickly enough. This caused temporary memory loss and some permanent nerve damage (neuropathy). Following the injection of these drugs, I had hallucinations for two days in which I saw filmy lilac colored webs in my hospital room, webs covering my husband, lace doilies on the wall, and a stairway to a throne room. Many unusual visions ran through my mind including golden threads being woven into cloth, animated flowers designed like cinnabar carvings, and lace wall hangings draped over staircases. Some of these mental images must have related to my career as a fiber artist. Other images were not so pleasant and I wanted to escape from the unreal world the hallucinations had created. My senses finally returned and I was able to concentrate on my husband, son, daughter-in-law and our dog. I wrote some of my thoughts in the hospital.

October 26, 1998

When closing my eyes, I think of Dennis, Tony and Aimee, and Hogan, our dog. Their pictures come into my mind; this was the first time in two days that I can actually visualize family pictures and home life. It is comforting and I feel it means the effects of ifosfamide are wearing off – I am approaching reality again. The bulb of a lovely lily must first lie under the soil, then burst into bloom, and bring pleasure and beauty. So must I. I must continuously give up dead cells so that new cells can grow. The dead cells are carried away and new cells promise life again. In life, there are periods of time in which one becomes overwhelmed with the world and the pace of life. During these times, one needs to re-evaluate what is most important. Old habits are discontinued and new, meaningful activities are substituted. These new activities restore life. With the disease of cancer, I have thought many times of the prospect of death. In my most frantic confused state, God came to my rescue and did not let me die; instead, He gave me a chance to live. It is like a new life for me – everything has changed. Dennis and I take time to love each other, to spend more time together, and to enjoy the beautiful creations of God. I appreciate the gift of this new life.

After the frozen stem cells were returned to my blood system, my platelets began to decrease to a dangerous level. A platelet transfusion that matched my blood composition, antibodies and leukocytes was needed. Platelets were located from the blood bank – six donors worldwide had the same composition as mine. This transfusion was given the next day, but I needed more. Our son was contacted, as he would likely have the same antigens as I have. His platelets were shipped to St. Louis from Omaha, but were not a perfect match. However, they were used twice; these transfusions gave me a boost until the platelet crisis improved. Another problem occurred indicating blood in my stools. An endoscopy was planned but then cancelled due to danger of damage to my esophagus from the procedure. Platelets were still too low to risk an injury that could cause bleeding. After thirty-three days in the hospital I was released to go home. My body resumed building bone marrow along with red and white blood cells.

After returning home, a home care nurse came every day for four weeks; she flushed my catheter and administered blood tests. I gained strength each day and entered the world of normality. A wheel chair made shopping easier. Daily walks helped to rebuild and maintain my strength. As I recovered, we began to plan an Elderhostel trip to Turkey for March of 1999. While my energy was limited, the recovery from the stem cell process was fairly quick.

Our son called on Thanksgiving eve and said he had broken two bones during a bike accident. We were quite concerned over his injury. We wanted to be with him, but did not think it wise to make the long trip to Omaha since I had just been released from the hospital. His arm healed after 2 steel plates were inserted in his arm and the bones were set.

My catheter that was used for the stem cell transplant procedure was removed before Christmas. Additional problems were addressed. A hearing test indicated I had lost some hearing in both ears and might need a hearing aid to allow me to hear high pitch sounds. In spite of medical problems, the Christmas holidays were joyful days filled with family and friends. It seemed to be a miracle that I could partake in active holiday events as I continued to regain strength.

1999

Living in Spite of Change.

An ice storm in January started 1999. Several days inside were a relaxing repose from the busy holidays. In mid-January, a hernia surgery was needed. During recuperation, I planned our trip to Turkey. My oncologist told me I could make the trip with no problems. I felt good. The weather turned into lovely 50-degree days permitting long afternoon walks. I completed several new art pieces and participated in an art show outside of Chicago.

In February, I had a gallium test (nuclear medicine). It involved radioactive material being injected into my vein to detect cancer in any part of my body. It revealed no large tumor masses; however, my CA-125 tumor marker was beginning to increase which was not good news. I felt good since I had not had chemotherapy for three months. An abundance of energy allowed me to remain active in artwork, in homemaking, and in social life. Many days were enjoyed at the lake studio as I worked and relaxed. I had days when I reflected on the disease that had changed my life.

February 20, 1999
I have been worried about my CA-125 going up and then heard of the death of another woman who had ovarian cancer. At times, I do become discouraged; I wish I could be completely cured of this dreadful disease. However, this "sentence" on my life has made me more aware of living in the present and has made me want to take advantage of each new day. I do not plan to spend all my time worrying about dying. We must all face our mortality – that is inevitable. Perhaps it is a gift to enjoy each day because there is no assurance of a set number of days remaining.

We went to Omaha to visit Tony and Aimee and to pick up an air-blast sprayer for the vineyard. This delightful city offers many events not found in our small rural community and we always enjoy our time there. We made our usual jaunt to the Old

Market with its brick streets and quaint shops. Gourmet coffee shops are located in just the right places for mid-morning and afternoon coffee. A day's itinerary included Chinese cuisine, a trip to the Farmers Market, and a performance of *My Fair Lady* accompanied by the Omaha Symphony.

In March, we took an enjoyable trip to Turkey for two weeks. Ephesus, Troy, Istanbul, Izmir, and Bursa were some of the more interesting cities we visited. The markets for ceramics, rugs, jewelry, and silk were exotic. We enjoyed the craftsmanship of painted ceramic ware, woven rugs, inlaid stonework, and exquisite silk scarves. Daily classes taught by local Turks gave us an insight into the local culture. We toured areas with classical Greek and Roman sculpture, visited areas where Paul lectured, and enjoyed the world famous, Grand Bazaar in Istanbul.

After the trip to Turkey, between March and June, life at home resumed to an active schedule of artwork for exhibition, family life, and a visit from Tony and Aimee. My cancer antigen continued to rise and I was beginning to be concerned that the stem cell transplant had not put my disease into remission.

April 14, 1999

I am disappointed that my antigen marker is continuing to rise. It was elevated to 57. I am hoping that my cancer had been obliterated by the high dose chemotherapy and stem cell transplant, which I had in October. There is a hopeless feeling again. Am I going to have to have chemotherapy again? If so, what can be given to me that is stronger than the chemicals I had before the transplant? Is this the final blow for me? The feeling of uncertainty permeates every day.

While I was concerned about the cancer antigen marker being increased, other scans were negative including a CAT scan and a bone marrow scan. Fractioning of the CA-125 was completed to identify the proteins involved in the antigen test. The results found an unidentified protein reacting with the test. It did not appear to be cancer. That was encouraging news.

The few art shows in which I participated during the spring and summer were enjoyable. A favorite was the Springfield, Illinois Old Capitol Art Show. My sister and I again took a day trip to Paducah to see the annual national quilt show. Quilts from all over the United States were on exhibit. Many quilts were of exquisite traditional design while others were artistic, contemporary statements. Not only was the quilt show enjoyable, the downtown area put on its finest display and featured shops selling quilts, quilt supplies, clothing, antiques, and crafts of all kinds. The city's quaint six-block downtown area is charming with its brick sidewalks, interesting shops, and elegant little diners.

I continued to feel good and was involved in many activities. In May, a reporter from a local channel in Paducah wanted to do a TV feature of my artwork. We spent a delightful afternoon together in the studio as I was interviewed. We talked about my weaving and collage work, and completed the photography for the short TV segment. In June, I walked in the Cancer Survivor's Relay for Life at the local junior college. I also exhibited a piece of my artwork at St. Louis University Hospital for the reception of stem cell transplant recipients. It was pleasant to again see my nurses who had attended to me during thirty-three days at the hospital the previous year. I was thankful to be able to attend this special celebration. In early summer, I enrolled in a quilting class in order to learn to make quilts. A family wedding in late June added to the busy summer events and presented an enjoyable time with our close family group. The wedding of our niece was a beautiful ceremony that combined traditions from both America and India.

In July, a PET scan (positive emission tomography) was administered. Radioactive glucose was injected into a vein and was attracted to any cancer cells in my body. Forty-five minutes were needed for the glucose to travel to different parts of my body. The scan included almost the entire body from one inch below the eyes to the knees. Cancer in small 2mm particles can be detected with this procedure. The results indicated that cancer might still be active in the left portion of my neck as well as in the lymph nodes of my liver. A CAT scan located cancer in the lymph nodes around the kidneys and liver (the porta hepatic area), the abdomen, and the neck. The stress of July was almost unbearable. We were totally consumed with my health problems, involvement with art shows, and sorrow over the death of our dog, Hogan.

By late July, my oncologist had enrolled me into a clinical trial, Phase 1, at St. Louis University Hospital. This fifth type of chemotherapy consisted of three drugs: docetaxel, carboplatin, and oral etoposide (VP-16) given every fifteen days. After the second treatment, my platelets dropped to 18 and a platelet transfusion was needed. A few days later, more platelets were required. My temperature began to rise and I was hospitalized for observation and a blood transfusion. The following dose of chemotherapy was decreased by 25% to lessen the drastic effects on my blood system. My oncologist informed me of the status of my disease and it was not particularly pleasant. I worried that the decreased amount of chemotherapy might increase the rate of the cancer growth. I was concerned that my tolerance of chemotherapy was beginning to fade. With all my fears and concerns, I attempted to find something positive from my oncologist's remarks.

September 1, 1999

My doctor explained that my cancer is a chronic disease and is not curable. It can be treated for a long time and is unlike lung cancer or some other types of the disease. The clinical trial in which I am involved was set up initially for lung cancer but was found to be effective for ovarian cancer as well. We are using as many options as are available to me and will eventually get to the end of the line of treatments currently on the market. On the other hand, he said that the only level of cancer that is at its limit is when a person is dead; then it can no longer grow. Cancer requires food to grow and of course cannot grow if not nourished. If no other drugs are on the market for treatment, highly experimental procedures are sometimes recommended if the patient has a lot of stamina to tolerate the treatment. For now, we continue to go down the line using less effective drugs that have good response and will continue using different drugs until we get to the end of the line.

On many occasions, I felt completely hopeless. Cancer had a way of controlling my life and thoughts. I wished there were some way I could rid myself of this dreadful disease and somehow escape from the clutch it had on my life.

Between each cycle of chemotherapy (each cycle composed of two treatments per month), I took advantage of my good days. Our son's new business was thriving and we enjoyed our visits with him. My quilt from the quilting class was put on a frame for the hand quilting process. I exhibited some of my work at the Cedarhurst Art Fair. Following each cycle of chemotherapy, I was admitted to the hospital for two or three units of platelets. Sometimes HLA (gamma globulin) was given to suppress the immune system from attacking the new platelets. Because of weakness, a wheel chair was often required in order to enjoy activities out of the home. A second PET scan revealed cancer still in my lymph nodes but no new cancer in any organ. There was an encouraging drop in my CA-125 antigen marker. The new treatment seemed to be effective.

With energy continually depleted due to continuous chemotherapy, I realized a need to simplify our lives. This included getting rid of items we did not need such as the boat at the lake, the studio piano, and some of my looms. On days when I felt good, we took excursions around Southern Illinois. We toured Heron Pond's wetlands, enjoyed the Ohio River lock and dam project at Olmsted, and drove through "Pumpkin Town" in Anna.

In October, I leased out the lake studio while contemplating selling it. It was a very special place, a place for creative work, solitude, and inspirational writing, but it was also an unnecessary item in our quest to simplify life.

Before Thanksgiving, our son was thinking of locating a building for retail space, warehouse facilities, and shipping area. The excitement of his business gave us something in which to be involved and kept our minds active in other aspects of life.

My car was developing some problems. Dennis drove me to the dealerships to look at new models but I was too weak to do a test drive. I eventually bought my car by phone and Dennis drove it home. For several days after purchasing the car, I was still not strong enough to drive it; this limited my freedom considerably.

Following the fourth cycle of the clinical trial, my oncologist was not pleased with the results of the treatment. The cancer had not been decreased 50% as expected; the antigen test again indicated an increase in the disease. The possibility of surgery in the porti hepatic area and the neck area was not an option due to the strategic location of the disease. A new treatment, doxorubicin, was started before the holidays. This was my sixth type of treatment. Fortunately it lacked the adverse side effects of the clinical trial and allowed me to partake in the feast of the Christmas holidays with a dinner party for my family, a long visit with Tony and Aimee, and a new puppy. In spite of this happy time, I had been "weepy" all week – tears came on Christmas Eve.

December 24, 1999
Perhaps I am finally facing the reality that I am not going to live very much longer. I am sad at the thought of leaving those I love. While I make an effort not to cry in the presence of others, I lost all control this afternoon as I was talking to Tony. I want to enjoy the progress of our son's growing business and be able to contribute to our family and society.

The last day of the year presented a most unusual situation – the weather at 55 degrees was perfect for a picnic in the woods. New Year's Eve was enjoyed as we watched *PBS Millennium Around the World*, including Times Square and Washington, D.C. festivities. It seemed an accomplishment to actually be a part of this end of the year celebration and the approaching new century.

2000

Planning for the Future.

The year began with mild weather and another picnic lunch in the backwoods on New Year's Day. The nice winter days kept my mind occupied allowing me to tolerate weekly chemotherapy.

The few treatments of doxorubicin were not as successful as my oncologist had anticipated. The cancer antigen marker indicated a rise to 533! This was the highest CA-125 reading since my initial surgery. I began to consider a pre-planned funeral. If time was limited, I wanted to make plans with the mortuary in order to alleviate the pain of decision-making for my husband and son. I became disheartened.

January 24, 2000

News of the antigen marker created such discouragement. Dennis attempted to encourage me by reminding me that we had been through this for over two years and that I was fortunate to still be alive. It is imperative that we enjoy every moment as we have tried to do the last thirty-two months. It is with awe that I have been able to withstand the trauma of multiple treatments; I am in awe of the human body and its ability to continue to function and repair under such conditions. God designed a spectacular machine. Mastered by the Creative hand, a spirit is generated which never dies. That spirit of man gives life meaning and hope of a purpose. Plans for a funeral, along with prepared statements, brought tears to my eyes. Life has been so good, so enjoyable; I don't want to leave right now. I want to be with my family. I fear that the cancer is growing too rapidly. I am afraid. There is a need to re-kindle the flame of faith that can give me hope. My acknowledgement of that which is Eternal has allowed me to trust my own instincts and to realize that hope is the core of well-being.

By the end of January, a seventh-line of chemotherapy was begun. This treatment utilized gemcitibine (Gemzar) and tamoxifen – having a 25-40% success rate for lowering cancer growth; daily oral doses of tamoxifen doubled chances of success. Side effects from this treatment were low platelets and decreased white blood cell counts. A Neupogen injection was needed for five days following each week's treatment. Neupogen increased the white blood cell growth. A Procrit injection was needed once-a-week to stimulate red blood cell growth. Dennis gave the shots to me at home; this proved to be more convenient than going to the doctor's office or hospital every day.

Side effects of Gemzar were less severe than previous treatments. I felt well enough throughout the year to participate in five art shows, continue family and social contacts, and attend a local Cancer Support group. These meetings once a month offered an opportunity to meet with other cancer survivors, share ideas on coping with cancer, discuss diet options, and receive spiritual support to address each day's problems. Special presentations were made which enhanced understanding of the special challenges faced by cancer survivors. A program presented by a pharmaceutical company clarified the option of morphine and opium pain treatment for the cancer patient who experiences unbearable pain. The information was helpful in relieving my fears of pain and informed me that drugs are available for pain management should that need arise.

The effects of two-and-a-half years of chemotherapy had taken a toll on my hearing, which necessitated a hearing aid. Peripheral neuropathy continued to be a problem with my hands and feet. These inconveniences did not interfere with our 40th wedding anniversary plans. We planted a blue spruce to commemorate our forty years together, took a cruise to Jamaica and Grand Cayman Islands and hosted a special wedding anniversary celebration with family and friends in our home with an evening of music, food, conversation, and renewed wedding vows.

By the end of March, we received good news that my disease was being treated aggressively with Gemzar. Results were encouraging; some areas of cancer had been reduced in size while other areas indicated a stable condition.

Joy over the improvement of my condition inspired us to take many outings with family and friends. On one occasion, we went to Cave-in-Rock State Park. The cave was as interesting as I remember it from childhood days when our family would spend a day in the park for fish fries. The riverboat offering fresh fish for sale reminded me of those days long ago when an excited little girl and her dad would board a boat to buy fresh river catfish for our dinner near the cave. The mounds of Ohio River carp and catfish had a pungent odor only experienced in such special places as the fish boat. Mom fried the fish and served the filets along with typical picnic fare on a flowered table cloth under a large shade tree.

I enjoyed keeping as busy as possible. However, I was not spending as much time with my artwork as I had done during all of my professional life. My artwork was not progressing as consistently as I expected; creative ideas had come to an abrupt halt. I was disappointed in myself.

March 11, 2000
I miss the challenge, the impetus to continuously be working on an idea, and the broad avenue in which to exhibit my work. While my mind desires one venue, my body restricts mobility and suppresses initiative.
It is frustrating.

During April through September, I participated in six art shows including Terre Haute, Chesterton, and Indianapolis, Indiana; Springfield, Illinois; and Milwaukee and Madison, Wisconsin. The shows differ one from another; most summer shows are outdoors while the early spring shows were often indoors. The

Terre Haute show was indoors and was an elegant evening of candlelight, art, food, and wine. Only ten artists were invited with about fifteen hundred guests present. Round tables dressed with white tablecloths, candle lanterns, and leaf florals surrounded by white netting graced the room. Candles glistened over square mirrors on each table. Overhead lighting cast a soft purple glow over the room. Artists' booths were highlighted with spotlights around the perimeters of the room. Green plants accented with tiny white lights added the final touch to the elegant aura of the room. A buffet of finger foods and wine were served to the guests and artists. Contrasting to this show, the outdoor show in Milwaukee, known as the Starving Artists show, had a completely different atmosphere. In this show, artists' displays were set up under tents outdoors. Patrons for the show lined up at the gate an hour before opening in order to have first choice for the art on display; they ran to various artists' displays to purchase their treasures. All art had to be priced $75 or under. Many artists reduced their prices drastically for this show.

Three weekly chemotherapy treatments each month were followed by one week off to recover. In April, the veins in my wrists and arms began to create problems; inflammation and swelling were the results of consistent weekly blood tests and chemotherapy infusions. In May, a portacath was implanted into my upper right chest. Blood tests were then taken directly from the port and chemotherapy was directed through the portacath. This device proved so convenient that I wished it had been implanted at the initial onset of chemotherapy. I would recommend other cancer patients talk to their oncologist about this at the beginning of their treatment. It made infusions and blood draws less painful; the veins in my arms were used only when the port could not be used.

Following the surgery for the portacath, I experienced some days of anxiety because the cancer antigen had again shown some increase. I became despondent and was also greatly disturbed over the death of a friend.

May 14, 2000
Today is Mother's Day. It was a "blue day" for me. My special card from Tony did not arrive; I am moody and a bit depressed. We attended a private memorial service for a friend who died after fighting breast cancer for several years. It was sad and contributed to my feelings of depression. I guess I am feeling sorry for myself while recovering from surgery, and attempting to cope with the events of the day.

An art show in mid-May around the Old Capitol in Springfield lifted my spirits. We stopped in Lebanon, Illinois before the show to attend a concert performed by a friend. The program included music of theater selections from 1900 to the present.

Following the Springfield show, my sisters and I had another overnight at the lake studio. The frequent visits from my sisters, along with their support, helped me maintain a positive attitude. My older sister and I celebrated our special birthdays; I was born on her third birthday, so we celebrate together if possible.

Spring was an active time with Dennis employed in helping with the 2000 census while I designed several framed wall quilts for art shows. The blueberry harvest was abundant; we picked several gallons of blueberries. For several weeks, the succulent berries found their way into pies, sauces, and our first blueberry wine.

All of July was consumed with making improvements at the lake studio. It was a painful decision for me to realize I must sell it. I loved the studio and the restful work atmosphere it provided. We painted walls, caulked molding, installed a new door, cleaned and waxed the floors, repaired the dock area, and pressure washed the house and garage. My energy level was low after treatments during the early part of the week; thus much of the work was done toward the end of the week when energy was more abundant.

Good news from my doctor indicated a stabilized cancer antigen and a decrease of 60% in cancer around my liver with no further advancement around my neck. I was elated. The weekly treatments were working well. Neupogen and Procrit injections were continued; these weekly injections allowed me to take my treatments on schedule if blood counts were elevated adequately.

Toward the end of the month, I received a letter from my oncologist indicating that he would no longer be continuing his practice because he was leaving the area. I depended upon his expert care and respected his decisions for me as I faced each crisis with my treatments. I was very sad to lose him as my doctor and wrote him a letter of appreciation for what he had done for me. I was referred to another oncologist and was quite happy with the patient/doctor relationship. It was to my benefit that I had two oncologists – one in my local area and the other at a research hospital in St. Louis. The local oncologist provided immediate care, regular office visits, and standard chemotherapy treatments; my oncology specialist, at St. Louis University Hospital, offered services in experimental treatments and clinical trials not available in smaller local areas. New drugs being researched were discussed with both oncologists. Through personal research and attentive involvement, I felt more in control of my disease. My two oncologists communicated with each other concerning the best decisions for my care.

Day trips with family or friends during June and July included St. Genevieve, Missouri and San Damiano in Southern Illinois. St. Genevieve is an early French settlement, which was inhabited by French Canadian settlers and entrepreneurs. The historical buildings reflect the lifestyle of the French settlers of that time. We also visited Fort Kaskaskia State Park where the Mississippi River changed courses and ran into the Kaskaskia River creating an island between the two rivers. The trip to San Damiano exposed us to a lovely villa retreat, neatly groomed grounds, and a peaceful environment for meetings and personal meditation; there were cabins overlooking the Ohio River for overnight accommodations. These peaceful places in Southern Illinois create an atmosphere of a quiet, relaxed environment where one can be released of life's stresses and can enjoy the beauty and serenity of nature.

Before harvest season from the garden and vineyard, we traveled to Omaha to assist Tony and Aimee with the renovation of a building for their *Premium Home and Garden* business. Dennis did repairs and cleaning while I washed and polished antique furniture for display cases. Following the trip, there were many weeks of labor in the vineyard; it required constant care with spraying several times before the grapes were harvested, thinning out grapes to assure that the final fruit was premium, and periodic mowing to rid the vineyard of weeds. I was not strong enough to help in the vineyard.

Late August presented some anxious moments as I began showing the lake studio to possible buyers. The studio had been my personal paradise for twelve years. I dreaded having to sell it. The second couple that came to look at it wanted it so strongly that they returned the next day with a down payment. We took pictures of the house for them, explained more details, and eventually signed the contract to sell the house. The final closing was in thirty days. I could not help but shed tears as I signed the agreement to sell the place that I loved so much; a place that had been such an enjoyable part of my life. I felt confident that the new owners would love the environment there as much as I had.

September 1, 2000
I find myself crying when I think of selling the studio. The decision to sell was necessary considering my health, but that decision also affects other decisions such as discontinuing my participation in art shows. I will no longer need to be aggressive and organized in creating multiple art works. This makes me feel as though I will accomplish nothing of value. I am feeling very sad because I want to spend more time at the studio before the closing date.

Early September yielded more grapes; Dennis was picking hundreds of pounds each day. I helped by selling some of them to local customers. He pressed juice for wine and stored it in barrels and we canned juice for the winter. He picked an additional five hundred pounds of Catawba, which is a sweet grape, good for making wine. An ad in the newspaper did not produce any new buyers, but familiar customers who wanted to make jelly continued to buy grapes. The wineries did not want small quantities; they preferred grapes by the ton. By the middle of September, I was very tired from grape harvest and was quite anxious of the closing date for the sale of my studio.

We made a quick trip to Omaha in mid-September. Our son's store was open to the public and we shared in his excitement of the new business adventure. We dined at a Middle Eastern restaurant, walked the Farmer's Market, and purchased fresh seafood at the local fish market. Back home, after the trip, we prepared the studio for the final closing date.

September 27, 2000

This is the day before closing the sale on the lake studio. We checked the house carefully and did some final cleaning. I had a few moments to sit on the dock, put my feet in the water for the last time, and reflect on the joy, peace, and relaxation this studio haven has offered me. I am thankful to have had this as part of an enjoyable life. I put fresh flowers in the kitchen and a welcome cake in the refrigerator, shed some tears, and left the house for the new owners, who will take possession tomorrow.

During the last quarter of the year, some major problems were beginning to surface; I had to address these early in the following year. Lymph nodes in my left shoulder were tender, cancer was beginning to grow in my neck area again, and pain in my lower right abdomen was becoming a problem. My appetite was decreasing which lead to overall weakness. It was an effort to accomplish anything I wanted to do or attempted to do.

We took several small trips to make life more interesting. Having something fun to do, in spite of the effort required, helped to keep my mind off of my health problems. One of the trips we thoroughly enjoyed was a two-day visit to Indiana. We stopped at New Harmony to see the old settlement, then proceeded to French Lick Springs. We stayed in a charming old hotel with a wrap-around veranda overlooking the elaborate gardens. A train ride into the Hoosier National Forest, a tour of New Baden Springs garden and hotel, and a delicious dinner at Montgomery Amish Village completed our tour. Another excursion took us to Wurst for the annual fest of wurst, kraut, and potatoes served in October. A jaunt through Fern Cliff State Park was an interesting short drive; another outing led to an overnight at a friend's house that overlooked the Mississippi River. It was a gathering of old high school friends who cherished friendship and time together.

December 11, 2000
My doctor has informed me of the necessity to change my chemotherapy regimen again. When the CA-125 antigen marker doubles from its lowest point with a particular chemotherapy, the treatment may no longer be effective. A type of chemotherapy used for breast cancer patients could possibly be used for ovarian cancer patients; however, my tissue sample revealed I did not have the gene necessary for this type of treatment. Another option would be necessary.

Having experienced many discouraging incidents, I decided not to allow this to ruin the festivities of the month. The holiday season began with the selection of our Christmas tree from the backwoods. Dennis dug up a small pine tree and potted it in a huge earthenware pot; the tree was just the right size for the kitchen. I decorated the little tree and we celebrated the holiday season with family dinners at home before flying to Omaha for Christmas.

While in Omaha with Tony and Aimee, I began to experience pain in my upper abdomen; I lost my appetite and noticed a discoloration of my urine and a change in bowel movements. Since I did not want to spoil Christmas for everyone, I masked my discomfort and we stayed in Omaha as planned. Upon returning home, I had a CAT scan which had been pre-scheduled weeks earlier. By that time, I was feeling poorly. I had lost six pounds and could not eat. On New Year's Eve, I was bedfast most of the day.

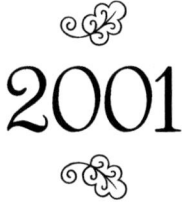

2001

The Will to Continue.

The year 2001was one of the most difficult I have had. I was very ill when the year arrived and new medical problems continued to present themselves throughout most of the year. I was hospitalized four times between January and August.

January 3, 2001

I did not have my regularly scheduled chemotherapy today because my doctor detected jaundice in my eyes. The CAT scan of late December reveals a tumor which is causing an obstruction in my bile duct; this obstruction causes the release of bile into the urine and stool. I was admitted to the hospital for an endoscopy. I am concerned about the procedure. The surgery is to be done by a friendly Pakistani gastroenterologist. We talked about the Middle East, the cuisine, and his family, while he explained the procedure to me. He told me he had been doing endo-scopies for twenty years. I feel comfortable with him as my doctor. He relieved my fears of bleeding during the procedure; the dose of vitamin K given me before the sur-gery would clot the blood until a cauterization would be done, if needed. I was very concerned about this matter since I have a low platelet count.

The endoscopy was done the next day. The procedure required about an hour, and a relaxant was administered. I lay on a table, face down; several pads were placed on my back with other devices attached to my body as I lay under a round machine. A screen registered what the doctor saw as a tube and small camera went down my throat. There was no pain – I was given a liquid to swallow that numbed my throat and esophagus. During the proce-dure, I was awake and could hear the doctor talk to the technician. The doctor expected to find a stone, but found none. A small stent was inserted into the bile duct to open the duct for drainage of bile. The following day, the procedure was again necessary because a larger stent had to be inserted. A few weeks following the endoscopy procedure, it was apparent that cancer was again active in the porta hepatic area near my liver. This required twenty-five radiation treatments to that area.

January 15, 2001
Due to the problem of the bile duct and radiation treatments, I have not had chemotherapy since mid-December. I am very anxious to start some kind of treatment soon! Gemzar is no longer working; some other drug must be used.

Radiation to the abdominal area around the porta hepatic was a delicate process. The liver, kidneys, and stomach were in danger of the radiation process. My radiation doctor said that side effects could result in damage to my right kidney; nausea and intestinal cramping could also result. If I did not undergo radiation, the enlarged lymph nodes around my liver could continue to expand; they would press against the bile ducts and the stent, causing the bile ducts to close and retain bile from the liver. There was so much with which to be concerned. Sometimes I longed for my parents – to share my concerns with them.

January 17, 2001
Today was my dad's birthday. He would be about 86 years old had he lived. He was such a wonderful father, so understanding and supportive. He had so much courage and determination. I am so fortunate to have had him as a father.

While taking radiation treatments, I stayed as busy as my energy allowed. I sketched, painted, visited friends, and practiced the piano; I had a goal to learn to play Dennis' favorite song, "Stardust" and one of my favorites "Nocturne in E♭" by Chopin.

I continued artwork, exhibited my work at the local Junior College, and hosted my high school reunion in our home.

In February, my oncologist started my eighth-line of chemotherapy. Taxotere and Arimidex were used but were not as effective as my doctor had hoped. These were discontinued until another chemical combination was initiated. Meanwhile, another problem surfaced.

Intense pain in my abdomen and intestines required pain medication; my doctor prescribed the Patch pain treatment. The Patch is a form of narcotic that consistently dispenses itself. The Patch is left on the skin for three days and is then replaced with another Patch in a different area. It can be used along with other pain medication such as Darvon. By mid March the pain was so intense that I was admitted to St. Louis University Hospital because of the discomfort, inability to take in food or water, no bowel movements and fatigue. An X-ray disclosed impaction and treatment was administered. After being released from the hospital a few days later, the pain continued and I was again unable to eat. I was readmitted to the hospital; a CAT scan and an upper GI series was done and another endoscopy was performed. The doctors suspected radiation damage to my small intestines. The endoscopy confirmed that suspicion; damage had been done and a huge ulcer was found in my stomach duodenum area. The days in the hospital were long and tiresome. Our 41st wedding anniversary was celebrated in the hospital with dinners from the hospital kitchen! Dennis was very tired from the 200-mile round-trip to St. Louis everyday. I remember that I made him promise to stop for coffee on the way home. Within six days, I was sent home with prescriptions for antibiotics, ulcer medication, an appetite enhancer, and a laxative. Chemotherapy had to be discontinued for several weeks due to my intestinal problem.

Two days after being released from the hospital, I noticed swelling in my left arm and neck. It extended to my legs, feet and face. A sonogram revealed no obstruction but a CAT scan indicated that the tumor in my neck had expanded into muscle area of my left armpit; this caused swollen lymph nodes and cut off the circulation of the lymphatic system in this area. To decrease the edema, I took water pills and used an elastic wrap on my arm until the swelling subsided. I also needed another fifteen radiation treatments for the large, recurring tumor in my neck. Radiation began in mid-April.

Weakness and general fatigue followed. My body had been through so many drastic changes in just three months. It was difficult to cope with so many problems at one time. It was traumatic to review my journals and re-live the pain, procedures, treatments, and decisions my doctors had to make for me. I am in awe of the trauma the human body can tolerate.

While recuperating from six days in the hospital and the swelling in my arm, we attended the Van Gogh exhibit in St. Louis. With the use of a wheelchair, I was able to enjoy the entire exhibit. I had limited energy, but was happy to be out participating in an event I enjoyed.

April 4, 2001
I am hoping God will renew my strength so that I can make some final plans involving power of attorney, financial planning, and talk with my minister concerning funeral format. I feel this is the time to do these things.

We attended to the need of establishing a power of attorney and medical directive for both of us and had those papers notarized. I arranged for a pre-planned funeral. I felt at ease having these things done. I wanted to spare Dennis the task of arranging my funeral. A visit from my minister helped to sooth anxieties I had in regard to dying. He encouraged me and consoled me in facing the daily trauma of a terminal illness.

In early April, an alternative chemotherapy regime was initiated. This was the ninth type of chemotherapy to which I had been exposed. It consisted of irinotecan (Camptozar), fluorouracil (5-FU), and leucovorin (Folinic Acid or FA), along with oral Arimidex in place of the tamoxifen. The new treatment caused fatigue and low blood counts. Neupogen and Procrit injections were again needed to stimulate blood cell growth. After every three or four weekly treatments each month, I had one week off. During this time, I was able to do some of the things I enjoyed.

April 7, 2001

A walk around the yard using my cane brought such joy in viewing the budding peach, apple and pear trees. Some of the trees are already leafed and flowering! The peach tree promises a few peaches. Dennis had transplanted the peonies to the front of the new fence. The irises are up and the anemones in periwinkle blue gloriously surround the big blue spruce. The blueberries are looking good – Dennis plans to transplant those to the South of the deck. We looked at the new plants coming back to life from last year – the lilies from bulbs mom had planted years ago on granny's grave, the iris, the magnolia bush, the burning bushes, peonies, hostas, dusty miller, and the daffodils along the driveway. I cannot think of a time when I have ever experienced such a feeling of awe and happiness over all the flowers as I have today!

April 12, 2001

Today is my mother's birthday. I love you, Mom, and have missed you all these years.

My mother passed away in 1982. I wished to share with her the many experiences of my life. She was a good mother, always supportive and ready to do what needed to be done. How I longed to have her comfort me when I needed it most. I wanted to tell her all of my problems and experience again her complete understanding.

During April and May, the weeks rolled by quickly with many pleasant endeavors and experiences. I had several good days in which I designed a special art piece featuring women around the world. The American Cancer Society accepted 150 reproductions of my paper quilts as a donation for their various fund-raising drives in Southern Illinois. Tony and Aimee came to visit for a few days as Dennis finished pruning in the vineyard and anticipated a good grape harvest later in the year.

A day outing with my sister, Lola, and her husband took us to Elizabethtown where we enjoyed a fish dinner aboard the River Restaurant. Touring this charming Southern Illinois area, we saw the River Rose Inn and the historic Rose Hotel along the banks of the Ohio River. Just outside the small river town was a lovely, quaint garden called Gillin Cottage Gardens. A side trip to Golconda took us up the steep hill to view the old river mansion my parents once owned. The house was once called the "Judge Sloan House."

Toward the latter part of May, I was having severe stomach cramps again. I needed pain medication of both the Patch and Darvon to alleviate the discomfort. Previcid lessened the pain of my ulcer and Reglan aided in digestion. Otherwise, good news resulted from the fifteen radiation treatments I had taken; the walnut-size tumor in my neck had shrunk to almost nothing. Treatments of Camptozar seemed to be keeping my cancer growth under control. My oncologist indicated that other drugs such as ifosfamide or gemcitibine with slow daily release might possibly be used when current treatment was no longer effective. I was always receptive to information about other treatments. Keeping abreast of new chemotherapy drugs gave me hope.

June 5, 2001

This is a lazy spring morning, somewhat dark and cloudy when I awoke. I did not want to leave my bed, but Dennis had a delicious breakfast of a cheese-vegetable omelet, bagel, orange juice and coffee ready. It was very good. After breakfast, I retreated back to the bedroom to enjoy my second cup of coffee. My room is such a pleasant retreat. I love this room and the comfort it offers. It is comfortably decorated with two wicker chairs, a library table from my mother, a small desk, and my favorite piece of furniture: a wicker sleigh bed. During the spring and summer, the bed is covered with a quilt I made in 1999. The quilt is designed of soft beige, ecru, white, and tones of hickory. The summer curtains are flowing white panels that are casual and offer an overall soothing atmosphere. Above the library table, a large framed quilt design of the same colors as the bed quilt is displayed. Dennis named my art piece "Remember Me Tomorrow." This room has been my comfort and refuge these four years; it always brings pleasure and rejuvenation whenever I need a quiet place to relax and recover. Everyone needs such a place, a place of intimacy and solace. I change the décor from summer to winter by using a palate of darker, richer colors. Floral draperies of ecru, white, cream, burgundy and green dress the window in winter and match the bed pillows that are trimmed in the same dark burgundy brush fringe as the valance. A white brocade bed comforter is used for winter along with three hand-woven ecru and white throw pillows. The carpet is dark green, the color of earth's rich foothold. The winter room décor adds warmth while the summer dressing is light and airy.

The months of June and July were difficult; overall fatigue and abdominal pain permeated almost every day. When there was a reprieve from overwhelming tiredness and pain, I used small spurts of energy to plant an herb garden and a few flowers. We visited family members and enjoyed dinners on the patio when I felt good. Each day, however, required a long nap to restore my energy level so that I could do things I wanted to do. I managed to finish a small sofa quilt with machine stitching, but most days, I was too tired to do anything. A wheelchair was used for grocery shopping. On some days, everything – including reading the newspaper – was an effort. In spite of all the difficulty I was having, everyday was a gift.

June 11, 2001
Each day I have something else for which to be thankful. Today it was the fact that I have had another day to be with Dennis as his companion. He loves to know I am here. I know I am loved and I know the feeling of love for him. It is truly a blessing, a fortunate moment indeed, just to be alive – to love and be loved.

I pondered the many ways Dennis has shown his love for me, offering me emotional support along the way. He has been unfailingly supportive and encouraging. His display of affection for me and his acceptance of my bodily limitations have been continuously reassuring. When I have been overwhelmed with physical incompetence and am forced to take a passive role in activities we once enjoyed, he accepts those limitations and does not make me feel guilty for my inadequacies. When I am disappointed in myself for not being active in creative artwork, Dennis suggests other activities that I might do. He assures me of his understanding and relieves my concerns of the imperfections a debilitating disease creates.

I realized that the spouse of a wife who has cancer makes unlimited sacrifices for her care. He gives up his own plans and needs to be at constant and immediate disposal of the needs of his wife. He becomes an avenue of support by taking charge of chores, being chauffer, and managing the household. Many times, he finds himself alone without a consistent active companion and must make adjustments for his own physical and social needs. As he feels stress and anxiety for his loved one, he also is confronted with the importance of structuring a life that would help him live alone should that need arrive.

My spouse has been my major caregiver. He has truly sacrificed his time and interests for my well-being. He has done this willingly in a loving and caring way. His kindness, comfort, encouragement, and love over these four years have given me courage to endure the anxiety; the regimen of treatments; the overwhelming fatigue; and the peculiarities of this disease. His understanding care has given me hope and has contributed to a positive state-of-mind.

> **June 13, 2001**
> We took a pleasant walk through the vineyard; the Concord grapes are looking good except for some spots of what is called "black rot" and a bit of fungus. We rested on the bench under the tree near the vineyard. It was enjoyable, beautiful, and peaceful. We are so fortunate to have this happy time together.

On one of my good days in June, my younger sister and I took an overnight trip to a lazy little town along the Ohio River; we stayed at a Bed and Breakfast accommodation overlooking the lovely scenic view. We walked along the riverbank collecting driftwood and enjoyed a fresh fish dinner as we sat in a shelter overlooking the mighty Ohio. The next morning, we feasted on an outstanding gourmet breakfast at the inn. An entrée of quiche with sausages, potatoes and a bagel were served along with trays of pastries, fresh fruit in crystal stemware, and orange juice. Our morning was completed with a tour of a perennial garden and a visit to an art gallery; the afternoon included meeting our other sister at a quaint historic town down the river. Again, my older sister and I celebrated our birthdays together.

Special days occurred whenever I had good news concerning the condition of my disease. Those days were particularly welcomed in view of the difficult six months I had experienced.

June 20, 2001
I had very encouraging results from my CA-125 antigen
test. The marker was 162 last month and had decreased
to 29 this month. Thank you, God! It means the radiation
to my neck and the present chemotherapy have been
effective in reducing cancer growth.

The summer months were pleasant with tolerable summer
temperatures permitting many enjoyable evenings on our new flag-
stone patio that had been built earlier in June. We had dinner on the
patio when my energy allowed it. Each week's chemotherapy
seemed to leave me more tired than the last. I could not sleep
soundly the first two nights after treatment and the chemotherapy
played havoc with elimination, with both constipation and diarrhea
being problems at various times of the week.

July 9, 2001
I am so tired all the time; I have to make myself perform
even the smallest tasks. I wonder if I am serving some
purpose, as I do not have energy to do anything that
might be a noble endeavor. I keep laundry done and cook
a few quick meals. I know I am serving one purpose, to be
with Dennis. That makes life worth living. Hearing from
Tony and Aimee along with visits from them makes my life
more enjoyable.

The inability to be creative – to do something meaningful or
to accomplish a goal – troubled me. I needed a project that made
me feel I had a purpose. With Dennis's encouragement, I decided to
consolidate some of the writings from my journals.

As I read the daily journals I had kept, I had both pleasant
and unpleasant memories. Recalling the tremendous struggle for
life, while going through high dose chemotherapy and the stem cell
transplant, was a horrendous memory. On the other hand, I was in

awe as I read of the many enjoyable days and months in which I had been blessed with life and the opportunity to live it. Attitude played an important role in my well-being as I endeavored to make each day a special occasion. Through the many pages of my journals, I sensed that this medium had been my solace and had actually helped me overcome many of my problems. Keeping a journal was a means by which I could deal with each day on a personal basis. It was a way that I could talk to myself and rationalize part of what was happening to me emotionally, physically, and spiritually.

In mid-July, I experienced acute pain in my right abdomen. My oncologist was on vacation, so I contacted my primary care physician; I was promptly admitted to the local hospital. After being treated for impaction, fever persisted; additional tests were completed. Antibiotics were given to reduce my fever. Tests revealed an infected gall bladder along with some other problems. It was necessary to see a specialist in St. Louis and make plans for a gall bladder surgery. I was moved to intensive care, was given a blood transfusion and was immediately transferred to St. Louis University Hospital by ambulance. A Hyde scan of my gall bladder was completed and additional antibiotics were given to me for twelve days to decrease the infection. A sonogram disclosed a few small gallstones. While in the hospital (a total of sixteen days), time crept by slowly and painfully. Decisions had to be made, by several doctors, concerning the severity of the infection and the need of immediate surgery. I was very frightened as I waited for the decision of the required procedure.

July 27, 2001
Much anxiety has been experienced over these last few days; I am not sure whether the surgery will be done now or after the infection in my gall bladder has decreased. I must rely on strength and courage from God that I find within myself.

The doctors informed me of the need for immediate surgery, but the surgery schedule at St. Louis University Hospital was full; I had to be transferred to St. Mary's for the procedure. The gall bladder surgery was done by incision rather than endoscopy. A duel surgery had been planned. It was to include rerouting of my bile duct into the small intestine to divert bile away from the lymph nodes near my liver. The stent that was installed early in the year was not removed. This part of the surgery was omitted since there was danger of infection from the gall bladder spreading to new incisions. Due to complications, what might have been an ordinary one-day endoscopy gall bladder surgery had turned into a 16-day, three hospital ordeal!

One's spiritual well-being becomes an important aspect of life, particularly for one who has a terminal illness. Mortality is certain and peace must be found in facing it. A conservative, fundamentalist religious doctrine during my childhood years instilled a fear of death and Hell. I had somehow failed to understand that God is a spirit of love, not fear. Fear is one of man's greatest enemies. I cannot think of God as my enemy, but as my greatest and closest spiritual companion. I have searched for comfort in God's grace.

August 9, 2001

I heard a poet's words concerning the use of language to express what one actually feels in his soul. His words of poetry were so expressive and so adeptly stated. It is a gift to be able to express joy, fear, trial, and one's appreciation of nature in such powerful prose. The poet felt that God gives the greatest blessings and opportunities to those going through episodes of despair, of trial, and of challenge. I wonder if that includes me. These four-and-a-half years have been a renaissance for me.

As I thought about my two sisters, and attempted to describe their influence on me, I felt overwhelmingly grateful for the happiness and inspiration they have brought to me. Without their love and friendship, my problems would be much more difficult to face. Because of my encounter with cancer, we have become closer, we have spent quality time together, we have confided our most heartfelt concerns, and we have gained an appreciation for our special friendship as sisters.

After a visit from my younger sister, Kasey, I wrote a long letter to her describing her infectious, invigorating spirit. After the storm, she is like the little bird; she is back out there reaping from life's bounty. She can see the effects of the storm, but catches its new fresh opportunities. She sees the fallen tree as welcomed firewood to keep someone warm. She faces each day with a fresh approach as her life reflects the exuberance she feels in expressing who she is and what she is about. A new day is another chance to see what nature has presented – some fresh blackberries, a little bird nest in the gutter, a new flower that has opened its petals, a succulent tomato on the vine, a cache of pecans under a tree, or the pattern of colored clouds from the setting sun. Never does a day end without some joy in living. Her life is a perpetual collage that continues to develop from life experiences. She respects and appreciates quiet moments alone in which she can reflect on her life, enjoy moments of solitude, and look inside to make contact with her inner self. There she finds a certain peace, an unexplained comfort, and contentment in searching deeply within. In this, she may feel God – the core of all natural things, the author of all thought and creativity. This saturation of strength, of fullness, of wholeness presents a mirror to reflect God in us, to exemplify beauty and grace, and to give back to others a portion of one's self. A sister such as this has been a powerful influence on me during our years of sisterhood.

My older sister, Lola, on whose third birthday I was born, has the fortitude of a saint. In spite of countless medical problems and family tribulations, she exhibits strength and spirit that allows her to face each day with great vigor and courage. Her determination in doing what is right is never compromised. She is analytical and searches for the appropriate response to each problem she faces. Her intuition toward those in need is unexplainable. Her storehouse of love, kindness and generosity are inexhaustible and her ability to forgive is exceptional. She truly shares herself with others in acts of friendship and love. It is from God that she claims her strength and remarkable fortitude, and it is through her belief in the Creator that her life radiates love and compassion for those around her. Her vitality and spirit have influenced my life and have provided me with encouragement during my darkest hours.

Somehow, my sisters and the beauty of nature always made the day seem brighter. Following chemotherapy, many mornings opened slowly with the strength to do very little other than praise the new day whether sunny or rainy. I sat outside on the deck to enjoy nature or simply rested a few extra moments in bed.

August 24, 2001

I am slow and lethargic this morning with no energy to do anything except enjoy a new day. It is a lazy Saturday morning which makes waking up gently seem particularly pleasing. The thunder outside my window may preclude rain – I hope so because I enjoy viewing the gentle rain, flowing down like pepper from a shaker. The rain has come now; it started as tears drizzling lazily down the window panes, then as torrents of gushing water, running uncontrollably down, cleansing the glass and working out its aggression as it pounded the window casing. Later it subsided and a slow show of drips moved gently, vertically, as it ran the length of the window. Viewing the process of rain is entertaining, as are other wondrous acts of nature.

Early September started the grape harvest. Dennis picked all the grapes within a few days. The harvest was small due to the frost in late April. The small yield was a big disappointment for Dennis since he had worked so diligently in the vineyard all year. I felt sorry for him and wished that the yield could have been more rewarding for his intensive effort. Disappointments were disturbing, but we immediately started looking forward to the possibilities of next year. Other unpleasant catastrophes were not as easy to rationalize.

September 11, 2001
This is a day of horror! Two hijacked planes crashed into the World Trade Center in New York. Later, a third plane crashed into the Pentagon and still another, possibly headed toward Camp David, crashed in Pennsylvania. It is a day of sorrow and awe. There has been so much destruction and loss of life caused by terrorists. My heart aches for those who have lost family members and loved ones. I am at a loss for words to describe the sadness I feel today.

September 14, 2001
The gloom of the past week seems to permeate everyone's thoughts. There is anxiety about a possible war, America's economy, and all the lives lost. It is depressing. My friend, Carolyn, sent an inspirational book to me "Grace for the Moment" by Max Lucado. This is certainly the time for grace, encouragement, faith, and for belief in God. The spirit of grace, righteousness, and correct decision-making is most necessary now.

From September through December, consistent chemotherapy of Camptozar treatments were taken for four weeks, one each week. A restoration period of two weeks followed before the next cycle began. A CBC blood test was required every week along with other blood tests every four to six weeks. Coumadin (a blood thinner) was adjusted according to the weekly PT blood test results. Neupogen shots were again taken for five days following chemotherapy and a Procrit shot was given to me each day that I had treatments. CAT scans of my neck, chest, abdomen, and pelvic were done approximately every three months. The latest results had indicated no new tumors in the neck and no increase in the size of the tumor in my abdomen. This was good news because it indicated that the chemotherapy regimen had been successful in keeping the cancer growth under control. This would change if the cancer cells built up immunity to this particular chemotherapy regimen.

Fatigue and inability to do household chores ruled each day. It was an effort to do the smallest task; taking a shower each evening was exhausting. Much of the fatigue occurred the day after chemotherapy and a few days before my next treatment. The nadir period is the name given to the time when the blood counts are the lowest. Several months were required to heal from the gall bladder surgery. Coupled with chemotherapy, my body had a big load to bear in recuperation. During days when I felt like doing something, we attended a concert, visited with my sisters, worked on a project together, or attended church. I worked consistently compiling notes from my journals into memoirs concerning living with cancer.

September 30, 2001
Dennis and I had a long discussion pertaining to the reason why I have been given this extra time to live. I questioned, "Is it because there is still something for me to do? Is there something more to accomplish? Is there something to finish?" I don't feel a calling to do any one special thing. I have lost some confidence in myself because of reduced energy level. I have lost the vigorous feeling of initiative and motivation. I don't believe in myself as I once did. I need Dennis to help me through rough times and to keep me inspired. He is like a father sometimes – one who always picks me up when I fall; one

who gathers me into his arms and holds me up until strength returns; like God who carries me through my darkest hours when I know not whom or where I am; like God who will never forsake me or leave me hopelessly alone. I am so thankful to have Dennis who takes care of my physical presence and God who takes care of my spiritual existence.

Autumn was the designated time for Dennis to transplant blueberries from the front yard to the backyard South of the deck. Strawberries were transplanted in the new garden space. Pumpkins were picked and stored for pies, soup, bread, and casseroles. Unseasonably warm temperatures required lawn mowing into late November and gave us many extra days of enjoyable weather out doors. Inside chores included cleaning the windows and replacing the summer curtains with winter draperies.

October 3, 2001
It's autumn now and I enjoy watching the dried, crumpled grape leaves tumble across the grass. The chestnut tree to the South of the deck stands gloriously, glistening in the sun and waving its colorful rusty red leaves. I love fall. It is one of God's gifts to mankind, particularly in our part of the Midwest on this side of the globe. I also enjoy the four seasons and respect the beauties and difficulties of each. Autumn seems to be perfect while winter in some areas is unbearably cold, spring sometimes has too much rain and summer can be a scorcher. Soon the frost will rest upon the few pumpkins remaining in the field and it will be time to stay indoors to enjoy winter's bounty of pumpkin pie, chili, and a pot of vegetable beef stew.

I had several good days during the fall season. Treatments on a regular uninterrupted schedule allowed me to plan activities during those days when I had energy. Any health-related accident had to be treated immediately to avoid more serious problems in the future. A severe laceration to my finger had to be nursed carefully for several weeks since chemotherapy patients have lower blood counts and are more susceptible to infection.

October 7, 2001
Disturbing news today indicated that the United States had started bombing Afghanistan. This is a serious situation and quite frightening. I pray our nation will make the correct response in this situation.

October 17, 2001
Tonight we viewed our slides from Afghanistan. The slides bring back a lot of memories from the mid-60's when we were Peace Corps Volunteers in Afghanistan. We have visited many countries, observed a variety of interesting cultures, and experienced many adventures that now seem unreal. We enjoyed the Afghan culture of colorful gardens, exotic Persian carpets and succulent rice dishes in a country filled with diversified tribal groups. Thirty-five years ago, Afghanistan was enjoying a time of peace with a king and a stable government. Today, after almost thirty years of turmoil, it is a country devastated by war, hunger, poverty, and lack of a stable government.

Late October was occupied with chores such as bringing plants indoors for winter, rooting coleus in water and cleaning up the outdoor deck and patio. Dennis spent much time in the vineyard pulling bull canes from the grapevines; he shaped these long twenty-foot canes into grape vine wreaths and a beautiful cone-shaped tree. I decorated the small tree with flowers, grapevine leaves, and a variety of pods and pinecones. It worked up beautifully and became our Christmas tree displayed on the grand piano for the holiday season.

We ate breakfast at a favorite restaurant once a week, usually on Mondays following my blood test at the hospital. On one occasion, we had a delightful visitor walk over to our table.

October 27, 2001
While having breakfast, a darling little lady with a smile on her face approached our table to say "hello." She said she just loved to see couples out having breakfast together. She wanted to greet us and in the process told us she had lost her husband about nine years ago and that she missed him. She was still living alone, doing her own lawn work, and canning peaches and apples. She was carefully dressed and was delightfully charming. She was 97 years old! Meeting this darling little lady was a memory I have cherished. She was an inspiration to me.

While a few pleasant days helped to keep my attitude positive, continuous chemotherapy on a weekly basis had taken a toll on my energy level and initiative. My blood pressure was consistently low, diarrhea was a problem, and potassium tablets were needed. This medication was added to my already bulging list of daily medications. One or two naps a day were a necessity in order to make it through the day. I became very discouraged.

October 30, 2001
My quality of life seems to be decreasing considerably. I am so tired I cannot enjoy the things I used to love to do.

During November, we processed several pumpkins for our favorite dishes. Pulp was scooped out of the oven-baked pumpkins, processed in the food processor and then frozen. During the next few weeks, the aroma of freshly baked pumpkin pie with plenty of cinnamon, pumpkin nut bread with spices and raisins, and pumpkin casserole with ham and potatoes emanated from the kitchen. All of these culinary delights made pumpkin processing worthwhile.

It was important to remain active, partake in some physical activity each day, continue frequent contacts with friends, and include social events in our schedule. We attended a concert at the local college and had family contacts frequently. In spite of my efforts to enjoy each event, constant fatigue was apparent each day and dampened the joy of every social gathering. On many days, it was difficult to prepare even a simple dinner or keep light daily chores done. With no energy, I felt helpless and useless. Each day was a struggle and each day I hoped to "feel better" so that we could travel to Omaha to be with Tony and Aimee for Christmas.

My chemotherapy schedule was considered before planning an early Thanksgiving dinner with my sister Kasey and an early Christmas gathering with both sisters. Since the chemotherapy drugs affected my appetite, we carefully chose a day when I was able to enjoy the festive food. Plans for the holidays were made to include those special moments that make Christmas the most important family affair of the year.

November 26, 2001
I had a slow start this morning with limited energy. During the afternoon, we did some Christmas shopping at the mall. Dennis took the wheelchair for me; allowed me to shop without getting too tired. I wrapped presents tonight while listening to Christmas music. It was a pleasant day. Thank you God, for these moments when I feel good and can enjoy life.

Preparation for Christmas was done as easily as possible; I planned a Sunday gathering for my family, made cookies, finished decorating, and addressed Christmas cards. The wines from the grapes needed to be tested and bottled before the holidays. Dennis asked me to critique each of the wines he had made.

December 6, 2001
It was rainy today, and was an opportune time to retreat to the basement to sample the quality of some of the new wines Dennis had made this past year. I analyzed four types of wine, judging each for color, clarity, legs, bouquet, and taste. All were evaluated on a scale A to E. I gave scores of A, B, or C on all four; none were bad wines, in fact, they were all fairly good.

The month of December offered a variety of Christmas displays, pageants, musicals, craft shows, and small extravaganzas. We took a drive-through tour of a special holiday light display and participated in a local craft show at the university near us. It was a satisfying experience to be out with others while celebrating the Christmas spirit. The desire to be part of the beauty of Christmas prevailed over my health problems. We left for Omaha in mid-December and were with Tony and Aimee for the holidays. Daily Neupogen shots were taken at the University of Nebraska Medical Center. I was grateful to have another year with my family during this special time of year and to face no additional major health problems while in Omaha.

2002

The Gift of Time.

As the New Year arrived, I reflected back on the previous year and what it had revealed. It had not been a pleasant year in many respects. I had been hospitalized four times, endured continuous chemotherapy treatments, had twenty-five radiation treatments to my abdomen and fifteen to my neck; I had a stent installed in the bile duct, suffered from an ulcer in my stomach, and had a problematic gall bladder surgery. In addition to health problems, the news on the world scene with terrorist activities further contributed to a year of gloom. Faith that "tomorrow would be better" and that "this too shall pass" kept me encouraged. In spite of all, life went on. Happiness was found in the blessing of life itself. Pleasures came in small packages and were accepted graciously.

The months of January and February were typical of long winter days and a hopeful attitude of getting organized before spring. The weather was mild and agreeable for Dennis's winter pruning. I made an effort to become inspired by a quilt design book one of my sisters had given to me; I sat at the computer typing my memoirs and made a presentation of several of my paper quilt prints to the church for the fellowship hall. By mid February, Dennis had dug two hundred and ten postholes in the vineyard; these were later filled with gravel, topsoil, and finally a grape vine cutting or a new plant.

In late February, Tony and Aimee came to visit and to escape the frigid temperatures of Omaha. Southern Illinois is much warmer than the winter weather to which they are accustomed. They spent a lot of time outdoors enjoying the mild weather and watching their dog, Mozart, and our dog, Cleo, run and play at will over eighteen acres of lawn, vineyard, and woods. Tony cooked salmon steaks on slabs of cedar outside one evening. The delicious aroma filled the crisp cool air around the outdoor grill; we bundled up and enjoyed the fire pit after dinner on that incredibly clear night with stars so bright and beautiful.

In early March, my CA-125 had dropped to 33! That was

within a normal range. The Camptozar treatments that I had been taking for eleven months had worked well; my CAT scans showed no new tumors. We were so happy with that news. I still needed to continue weekly chemotherapy sessions, however; they were aggressive and had a variety of usual side effects. I was constantly tired and weak, had bowel problems, stomach pain and some intestinal cramping. There were a few days each month when I felt strong enough to enjoy the outdoor world – that had begun to mean anything outside of my immediate, comfortable and safe home environment! We celebrated our 42nd wedding anniversary by attending an art exhibit and artists' reception at Dunn Richmond Center in Carbondale. The show included one of my art pieces titled "Mosaic of Women."

While organizing stored treasures of photo albums, greeting cards, and mementos, I came across several letters from my parents. I remembered their fortitude as they journeyed through life dealing with their various problems. I found inspiration in some of their comments. A particularly loving letter from my mother exposed her views on working together for a happy, healthy, successful marriage. Other letters were from my father who suffered from grave health problems. Written only a few weeks before he died, he fervently wrote of the beautiful flowers he had planted in the yard, the hunting trips he had taken, the many projects in which he was involved, and a note concerning what he was planning for tomorrow. His letters exposed his thankfulness for life – he was "happy to be alive and to enjoy the wonderful world which God has made for us." In spite of his severe illness, his letters revealed an enthusiastic passion for life, a thankful attitude for it, and a desire to live life in its entirety. As I re-read the letters, I felt sure that he was telling me that he was not giving up but was accepting with thanksgiving and reacting with pleasure to the time that remained.

In early spring, I helped Dennis display and sell pruning tools at a grape growers meeting. He planted an early garden and took a wine-making class at a local college. I exhibited an art piece in a local art festival and won a second-place cash award in the collage category. For our birthday, my sister and I were treated to a special birthday celebration hosted by our younger sister who had arranged a Bed and Breakfast overnight at Annie's Cottage in Cape Girardeau, Illinois. The occasion included a special picnic supper at Annie's cottage, a tour around the old part of the city's antique district, lunch at an Italian restaurant and a visit to a popular rose garden. Later in the spring, Dennis and I took a trip to visit Tony and Aimee to see their new home. My strength was always limited, often forcing me to omit or cancel activities we had planned; I spent half of each day in bed or lying on the sofa. I felt myself slipping into a slight depression.

The loss of an acquaintance I had met in the infusion room at the doctor's office did not aid my already broken spirit. This delightful woman had been a nurse. She was so entertaining with her marvelous sense of humor and her charming mannerisms. I liked her and enjoyed her attitude of amusement. We often had chemotherapy on the same day, sitting side-by-side. I knew I would miss her. Her memorial service was thought provoking as I learned of the many services she had performed for her church and for nursing ministries. Notes in my journal expressed a desire that I wished my life had been as great as hers in terms of service to God and to mankind.

The regimen of chemotherapy once-a-week for three weeks followed by two weeks off had become tiresome. I dreaded my weekly sessions that caused so much fatigue week after week. I often fell asleep in the chair while the drugs were being infused. It was normal to have an upset stomach and decreased appetite for a several days following infusion. I disliked having to go to the hospital each day for a Neupogen injection especially on days when I did not feel like getting out of bed to attend to this daily ritual. My health insurance would no longer pay for the injections if Dennis gave them to me within the convenience of our home; the shots had to be taken at the hospital or doctor's office. If my temperature reached 100.5 degrees, as it did on several occasions, I had to immediately go to ER for antibiotics. At times, I felt that a sentence was upon me.

May 2, 2002
It is sometimes difficult to accept the consequences of this terrible disease. It seems I wait for death – like a shadow following me that will catch up with me. I hope that I am not in pain in my final days and can die peacefully with Dennis by my side, holding my hand.

After five years of coping with the daily problems that cancer creates, I found that I was losing some of the enthusiastic hope I had entertained years earlier; I realized I had to accept whatever happened. I was disappointed in myself that this attitude had made itself apparent!

Ovarian cancer may strike one of every fifty-five women. If detected early, it may be treated, leaving the patient cancer-free. In the latter stages of the disease (Stage IV, of which I had been diagnosed), the prognosis is not as positive. The disease, however, can be treated for a long time with the patient sometimes going into remission for a few months or possibly a year. My disease had never gone into remission. There were no disease-free intervals. Consistent chemotherapy was necessary to destroy cancer cells as they existed, or new cells that were being created. As cells were terminated, the tumor would shrink. When the current chemotherapy drugs were no longer effective, cancer cells would start growing again, sometimes in another area. I knew that I would most likely never be completely well again. I was resigned to the fact that I would neither be free of cancer or the chemotherapy treatments. It was my daily challenge to live with this phase of my life and to make it as significant as possible. I continued to manage anemia that made household tasks more difficult; chores were often left undone, meals were sparse, and I found myself going to bed to get through many days.

June 19, 2002
I don't like this state of debilitation. My life seems useless, uninteresting and boring. I am not contributing to society or accomplishing anything worthwhile. Dennis' life, on the other hand, is productive and determined. He is my hero who continually holds up an ideal for me. He works faithfully in his vineyard, creating a lovely place, or simply acts as a caretaker of one of God's wonders. He works diligently without monetary reward and accomplishes something of value each day. His quest for knowledge is insatiable. How I admire him and his efforts! He is truly a good person. I am in a state of inadequacy... but must do what I can do. Life must go on to the end, and hopefully I can be pleased with what I have been able to accomplish in the short span of a lifetime.

In early May, my left side had become painful; the cancer antigen indicated an increase in cancer cells. A PET scan in July revealed a tumor deep within my abdomen, probably within my lymph nodes. My oncologist in St. Louis laid out a new plan for chemotherapy treatments and radiation since the cancer was no longer responding to the previous regimen of Camptozar. By the end of July I was again taking radiation; I had some concern for kidney damage – this time my left kidney was near the radiation area. That was a chance I had to take. The previous year, radiation was done close to my right kidney.

Dennis worked faithfully in the vineyard fighting off the ravaging birds by using netting to protect the grapes. He had plans to sell the grapes to a winery. I completed another seventeen radiation treatments and started on the tenth chemotherapy plan; this time, methotrexate tablets and Zoladex hormone implants were used. My tumor marker had more than doubled again. Tony was concerned about my health and decided to come home for a short visit. His visit cheered me up as I watched father and son picking early grapes and pressing out the juice.

We were saddened by news that one of our best friends had been diagnosed with lung cancer. Our hearts were heavy with concern and anxiety for him and for his wife as they faced the agony that this disease creates. It was as though we were encountering my ordeal all over again. I thought of all the discomfort he would have to endure – the chemotherapy, the weekly blood tests, and the daily Neupogen injections. We attempted to be helpful with information and encouragement.

By late August, the birds had stripped the vineyard. Only the grapes covered by netting were saved from the robins and starlings. I walked down one row of the vineyard to view the lovely Catawba grapes before the birds feasted on those also. The exceedingly hot, dry summer increased the amount of birds in our area. They were looking for food wherever it could be found. Dennis managed to harvest about a thousand pounds of grapes to sell to a wine maker and salvaged a few hundred pounds for himself. He pressed the grapes into seventy gallons of juice.

In early September, I encountered more complications; lung pain, stomach distress, a rash, and dangerously low platelets of 6. The normal range for platelets is 150-400. I was hospitalized for six days for platelet and blood transfusions and Neumega injections to enhance platelet growth. I was released from the hospital when my platelets reached 100. The problems may have been due to methotrexate; my oncologist reduced the dosage to prevent further decrease in platelets. My CA-125 had been reduced from 269 to 90 probably due to the radiation treatments. We were happy to have some good news.

We enjoyed an Audubon exhibit at the state museum gallery at Whittington and an antique show in McLeansboro, Illinois with the aid of my wheelchair. The new chemotherapy plan did not cause as much weakness as the previous regimen. It was again pleasant to be out with friends attending some of the interesting events in Southern Illinois. We stopped at the quaint Vulture Fest in Makanda and viewed nature displays in the tourist center of Giant City State Park. October was an enjoyable month. In addition to all of the outings, I felt well enough to clean windows, have some dental work done, and shop on my own at the mall. Dennis felt more at ease since I did not need his constant care. He attended some lectures on viticulture at SIU and participated in a grape growers conference at Mt. Vernon. He organized tools and equipment for storage in a carport he had built near the barn. I was glad he had time to do some of the things he wanted to do and was elated that I was able to do something each day also. I could feel myself returning to the "I can" mode and it was gratifying! I compiled a book of recipes to give to Tony; many were his favorites from childhood. I hand-wrote each recipe with explicit instructions for some of the more difficult Persian dishes.

November 17, 2002

The message at church this morning concerned using one's talents to capacity – doing the best one can do within the perimeters of talents given to that individual. There is so much I wish I had done in using mine. I wished I had worked harder, had been more disciplined in some areas – mainly music. I am pleased with much of my artwork, but not all of it. There is still time for me to work more diligently and to use my abilities to their fullest. I must make myself do it – at least try. But as Yoda says "We either do or we don't do – there is no try."

As the holiday season approached, Kasey invited me to attend an art show that included one of her first paintings. Our son phoned with exciting news that his three-year-old Internet business was being included in a feature article of *Inc.* Magazine. Lola and her husband were going through difficult times with health problems. Family activities and involvement kept us busy before we went to Omaha for Thanksgiving.

Before our holiday dinner, Tony and Aimee took us to see a delightful performance of A Christmas Carol at the Omaha Community Playhouse. The Old English delicacies of the season could not surpass the festive Thanksgiving feast Tony and Aimee prepared! A twenty-six pound turkey took center stage along with traditional side dishes and Tony's homemade dinner rolls. An elaborate tray of imported cheeses and sculptured apples started the meal. It was a special time together being thankful for the good things the year had brought us.

In early December, my cancer antigen marker was again elevated; it had increased to 106. My oncologist adjusted the amount of methotrexate again, this time increasing the amount of days that I took the drug. He was hoping this would lower the antigen count.

Sidelining medical problems, I decided to put up the Christmas tree and decorate it; I had not felt well enough to do so the two previous years. I had forgotten the joy of handling all the ornaments that brought back so many memories of past Christmases. It was particularly pleasant to sit by the softly lit tree in the early hours of the morning when I could not sleep.

Our annual "three-sisters" pre-Christmas dinner was not possible due to the increased health problems of my brother-in-law. All three sisters realized that the health problems of ourselves and of our companions sometime prevent many of the traditions to which we are so dedicated. Being with Tony and Aimee for the holidays was again in our plans. We traveled to Omaha.

Celebrating Christmas while operating a business is an event in itself! Tony and Aimee's *Premium Home and Garden* store was an active place to enjoy the holidays. The shelves were lined with beautiful gift items, housewares, gourmet foods, grilling supplies, sushi serving pieces, art, personal care products, and a selection of fine wines. The phones rang for on-line orders and customers walked the aisles of products selecting items as varied as a teapot to a cast iron doormat. Dennis and I joined the work force doing odd jobs in the store. He acted as a handyman who assembled boxes for daily shipments, took out the trash, and vacuumed the carpet. I put merchandise data receipts in numerical order ready for filing. We often ate lunch at the shipping room table in the back of the store. The annual Christmas party for the store took place at an Italian restaurant that served the food family style. Our active schedule did not prevent my usual afternoon rest. If need be, there was a sofa in the office upstairs. My weekly blood test was taken care of at the hospital. On Christmas Eve, we remained at the store throughout the day and enjoyed the excitement of last-minute shoppers who were searching for just the right gift item.

At 4 p.m. in the afternoon, the store was closed and our family Christmas Eve began. Tony prepared an elegantly seasoned ham complimented by Aimee's side dishes. All four of us stirred the pot that contained fruits, nuts, butter, flour, ginger and flavorings for Tony's homemade fruit cake – the collective stirring was a symbolic action for good luck, supposedly.

After dinner, we exchanged the many gifts that surrounded the Christmas tree on the hearth. I had wrapped an unexpected treasure for Tony – his grandfather's pocket watch attached to his great-grandfather's watch fob and chain. It had been one of my father's cherished possessions as it was a gift to him from my mother; it had become subsequently one of mine. For me, it symbolized a gift of time, somewhat. It seemed the appropriate moment to pass it on to Tony as a particularly meaningful symbol of time through four generations.

Christmas morning found the "stockings hung by the chimney with care..." – as always an orange and an apple were there, plus a lot of other goodies! Even Mozart enjoyed his stocking with dog cookies. After breakfast of ham and eggs, we changed our traditional Christmas Day from focusing on a festive dinner to going to the theater to see a movie. Upon arrival back home at 5 p.m., I started preparing the chicken and dumplings I had promised to cook for Christmas dinner. Tony and Dennis cut up the chicken while I mixed flour and eggs for dumplings. Surprise! I discovered there was not enough flour for dumplings! No problem – Dennis found a store open and solved that dilemma. By 7 p.m. the chicken and dumplings were ready to serve. Aimee's dessert of peppermint ice cream sandwiches completed our meal. We enjoyed a most memorable Christmas Day with time together being the best gift of all.

Another holiday season had come to an end with unique moments to record and remember. The year had presented its challenges but also had offered many rewards, the greatest of which included sharing another year with our family.

As I close my journals and reflect upon the previous five-and-a-half years, I acknowledge that it has been a difficult journey but it has given me an opportunity to examine my existence. I have learned to appreciate life and to respect it as I became aware of how precious and meaningful life can be. According to statistics, the five-year survival rate for patients with ovarian cancer, Stage IV is 5%. I do not know why I was spared but am grateful to have lived through this part of my life. When I was first diagnosed, the disease had metastasized to my liver and lymph nodes. Even with that knowledge, I had an underlying hope that my condition would improve. There was a possibility that the cancer would go into remission after initial surgery and several rounds of chemotherapy.

Over the next few years, my options included several different classes of chemotherapy drugs to control the disease; each drug or combination of drugs were used as long as they were effective or as long as my blood system could tolerate them. In addition to chemotherapy, I had been given eighty-two radiation treatments. While I was fortunate that these alternatives kept the cancer within control, my disease never went into remission. I recognized that ovarian cancer was part of my life and I must cope with it as such. As side effects from the various drugs began to create other health problems, life became more difficult and my quality of life became greatly diminished. I lost much of my self-esteem. Even hope sometimes turned to hopelessness as I analyzed the facts of the disease. I found it difficult, if not impossible, to concentrate on the gift of life during times of physical and emotional pain. I was disappointed in myself. I needed help in maintaining a will to live and tolerance to withstand each of the ten different chemotherapy regimens as they occurred. I obtained strength through my husband's constant encouragement, through the network of support from family and friends, and through my own spiritual beliefs.

My personal faith and Dennis's support gave me determination to confront life while facing incredible obstacles. The need to believe that the body can be spiritually whole without being physically whole calmed me during moments of trauma. Becoming whole, in spite of illness, is a product of one's faith. Spirituality involves a meaningful relationship to one's Creator – finding and experiencing well-being through one's belief in God. Through prayer, I have sought ideals that offer courage, strength, peace and comfort during moments of hopelessness. Positive thinking and believing in myself have given me a desire to embrace life. The daily love and encouragement from my husband, his counseling and his persuasion has kept me connected to life. He has given me an incentive to be and to interact. We have embraced love as eternal; this love has given me a purpose for being.

These challenging years have presented many rewards. My marriage has become intensely stronger and more meaningful. I have a greater closeness with my son. Relationships to my sisters have grown into a bond of friendship and trust. I have learned to evaluate myself and to focus on that which is possible. I experienced miracles through the wonders of medical science and many doctors whose expertise gave me extra time to enjoy my family. I have been given the opportunity to view life in a new light, to see beauty about me, and to appreciate the subtle pleasures of today.

When the time comes that treatment is no longer possible for my disease, I must accept the inevitable conclusion of my life; I hope I will be courageous and will accept that fact graciously, remembering with thanksgiving the rewarding life I have been allowed to experience as I look forward to eternal peace.

August 1, 2003

Looking back at the past six years, I am thankful for the opportunity to have lived and to have enjoyed time with my family. The rewards of the journey far outweigh the moments of despair. Current treatments of chemotherapy give me additional time to enjoy the blessings of life. Considering the advancing research in cancer treatments, I look forward with hope to the future. I encourage anyone with cancer to maintain a positive attitude and to trust in the possibilities of today and tomorrow. Life is worth living!

The prescription drugs/treatments and trademarked drug names listed in this book are the property of their respective companies and were prescribed by licensed physicians as part of a personalized cancer treatment program for Nina Davidson Arnold and as such may not be an effective treatment for other individuals.

Order Additional Copies of

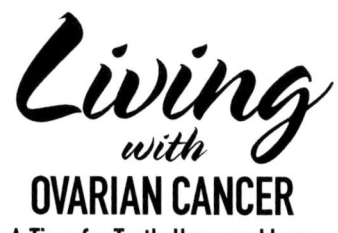

OVARIAN CANCER
A Time for Truth, Hope and Love

Send $12.00 for each copy (includes tax and postage) to:

Nina Davidson Arnold
Living with Ovarian Cancer
P.O. Box 51
Johnston City, IL 62951-0051

Number of copies: _____ x $12.00 = $ _____

Payment Options ☐ Check ☐ Money Order ☐ Cashier's Check

(Make payable to: Nina Davidson Arnold)

No cash or credit cards please. All sales are final.

Shipping Address _____

Name _____

Address 1 _____

Address 2 _____

City _____ State _____ Zip _____

Phone (_____) _____

Wholesale inquires welcome.